Medicine and Nazism

Daniel S. Nadav

Medicine and Nazism

Daniel S. Nadav

THE HEBREW UNIVERSITY MAGNES PRESS, JERUSALEM

Published by The Hebrew University Magnes Press
P. O. Box 39099, Jerusalem 91390, Fax 972-2-5660341
www.magnespress.co.il

Hard cover ISBN: 978-965-493-432-9
eBook ISBN: 978-965-493-433-6
Printed in Israel

In memory of my beloved mother

Edith Lowitsch
1913–2008

Contents

Prologue – *Non omnis moriar*

(Not everything is doomed to die)

Dr. Israel Milejkowski, the Head of the Public Health Department in the Warsaw *Judenrat*, concluded his introduction to the results of the Hunger Disease research with the Latin – "Non omnis moriar." Jewish physicians in the Warsaw Ghetto discussed this secret research report in the summer of 1942, just before many of them were dispatched to the gas chambers of Treblinka.

This act of defiance, along with maintaining an underground School of Medicine in the ghetto, was possibly the finest example of Jewish intellectual resistance in the medical realm during the Holocaust.

Still today, not enough is known of the efforts of Jewish doctors to uphold the tenets of medical ethics and help their brothers in need (and indeed others, such as the Gypsies in Auschwitz) in the face of death.[1] Both doctors and patients operated in what Primo Levi calls "the gray zones," left to them in the Nazi camps and ghettos.

My main motive in writing this book, appearing originally in Hebrew, was to unveil, in a concise fashion, the attitudes and activities of the victims themselves against impossible odds.

Additionally, after I had been teaching at the Tel Aviv Faculty of Medicine for many years without a satisfactory text on the subject, I wished to provide students at long last with an introductory book.

My Hebrew translation (1992) of Benno Müller-Hill's important book, **Murderous Science** (published originally in German in 1984), only partially served this purpose. Müller-Hill had bravely unmasked

---

1   See Etienne Lepicard's English review of my book in **Tel Aviver Jahrbuch für deutsche Geschichte**XXXVI (2008), pp. 358-361.

the participation of the German scientific establishment in the medical horrors of the Nazi period, but had hardly mentioned the deeds of Jewish physicians. Other excellent scientific publications such as the relatively recent companion book to the U.S. Holocaust Museum exhibition **Deadly Medicine** (2004), suffered from the same deficiency. This gap in our knowledge needed to be filled.

I have sought, however, not to "ghettoize" my account. Jews were not the only ones who suffered under the distorted Nazi Medicine. I have, therefore, tried to describe the effects of its criminal acts upon "ordinary Germans" as well. We should remember that the first 70,000 victims of the so-called "Euthanasia" program (1940-1941) were "Aryan" Germans. And up to a quarter of a million were murdered, even after the formal end of this action.

The origin of my Hebrew book was a series of 13 prestigious "Broadcast University" lectures sponsored by the Israel Ministry of Defense (MOD). The book based on these lectures, which appeared a short while later (2006), contained a new chapter devoted to "proper" medicine in the Third Reich, including its undoubted achievements in the struggle against cancer. My feeling was that a scientific book should not ignore the positive aspects of German medicine, even in the racist and totalitarian surroundings of Nazi Germany.

The brief text of the radio broadcasts (exactly 22 minutes per lecture!) dictated to a large extent the scope and appearance of the book that followed. No footnotes were necessary, and only a short selective bibliography, mainly in Hebrew, appeared at its end. Those constraints were relaxed somewhat in the English edition. A few notes were added and a brief bibliography in English and German was appended to each chapter. An effort was made, however, to preserve the survey-like character of the whole book, still intended to serve as an introduction for both students and educated people wishing to engage with an as yet neglected field of knowledge.

I have had the good fortune of enlisting my close friend, Elan Galper, to do the translation. Having studied medicine and taught English literature and history at Canadian and Israeli universities, he seemed an ideal man for the task. A modest stipend from the Yoran Sznycer Fund of Tel Aviv University, directed by Prof. Dinah Porat, allowed us to realize the plan.

Many other friends and colleagues in Israel and abroad have lent a helping hand and allowed me to use some of their findings in the Hebrew book. I would like to thank them again in the English edition:

Prof. Gerhard Baader, Dr. Tzvia Balshan-Dvorjetski, Mr. Joel M. Bray, Dr. Nava Cohen, Advocate Jonah De Levie, Prof. Esti Dvorjetski, Dr. Rivka Elkin, Prof. Caris-Petra Heidel, Prof. Shmuel Kottek, Advocate Joel Levi, Prof. Benno Müller-Hill, Prof. Kurt Nemitz, Mrs. Miriam Offer, Prof. Avi Ohry, Dr. Judith Reifen-Ronen, Prof. Shmuel Reis, Dr. Yoram Sandhaus, Prof. Shaul Shasha, Dr. Tomi Spenser, Dr. Michal Unger and Prof. Henry Wasserman.

Yad Vashem, the Israeli Holocaust Memorial and Documentation Authority, accorded important help to me. A research fellowship from Yad Vashem enabled me to spend a whole semester in its archives in Jerusalem under the auspices and guidance of its International Institute. The Institute's Director, Prof. David Bankier, did everything possible to assist me in enriching the quality and quantity of the sources needed to write some of the chapters in the book. These resources were particularly useful in compiling the chapters dealing with the Jewish "prisoner-doctors" in Auschwitz and with the criminal medical experiments. I would also like to mention the good advice given me by Prof. Yehuda Bauer, Prof. Israel Gutman, and the Chief Historian of the Institute, Prof. Dan Michman. In addition, Yad Vashem put at my disposal most of the photographs used in this volume.

It should be said, however, that the views expressed in my book, concerning the "Medicalization of the Holocaust" for example, do not necessarily reflect those of Yad Vashem.

I want to thank Magnes Press and its General Manager, Mr. Hai Tsabar, for their splendid work. They did their best to maintain the high standards which made this academic Institution famous in the last eighty years.

The book is dedicated to the memory of my beloved mother, Edith Lowitsch [born Margolinski] (1913-2008), who witnessed the beginning of Nazi barbarism, but was fortunate enough to leave Germany for Palestine in 1935 together with my future father, Helmut Fuss.

Daniel S. Nadav
Ramat Gan, July 2009
(pardoph@netvision.net.il)

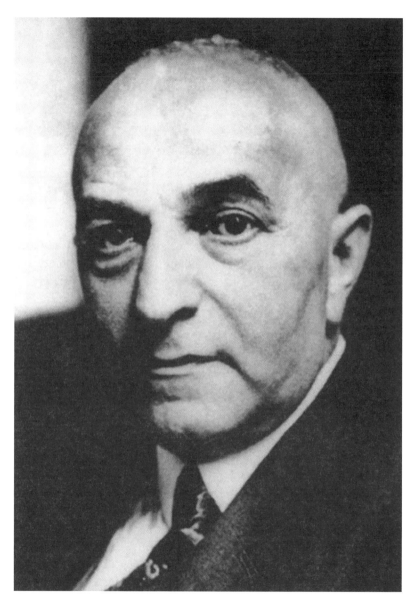

Dr. Julius Moses (1868–1942). Courtesy of AdsD, FES Germany.

Chapter 1

Medicine and Nazism

Introduction

In February 1932, a year prior to the Nazi rise to power in Germany, Dr. Julius Moses, a Jewish physician and a member of the German Reichstag,[1] published a series of warnings. These were heeded by very few at the time, possibly because the journal in which they appeared (and which Moses himself edited), **Der Kassenarzt,** had such a limited circulation. The German public, including the Jewish community, did not yet regard Hitler and his Nazi Party as a real impending danger.

Moses wrote:

> "Everything hitherto considered a supreme precept of medicine: the treating of the ill without regard to their belonging to one 'race' or to another, dealing with all patients according to the principles of equity, aiding everybody and relieving their pains – all of this is not considered worthy in the eyes of the National-Socialists [Nazis]. On the contrary: in their desire to wage a total war against the 'valueless' people of all sorts, and in particular the hopelessly ill, and to be rid of them [...] those patients having little chance of recovery are destined for annihilation, and the physician, in particular, would be appointed to this task."

In the last incisive sentence, Dr. Moses declared: "The physician would become a murderer!"

Despite his prophetic words, and the urgings of his eldest son, Dr. Moses refused to leave Germany for Palestine. He was finally

---

1   Daniel S. Nadav. **Julius Moses (1868-1942) und die Politik der Sozialhygiene in Deutschland.** Gerlingen: Bleicher, 1985.

dispatched by the Nazis to the Theresienstadt Ghetto, where he died of pneumonia in September 1942. The year before, however, he still managed to receive information, through his contacts, of the mass murder of Jews by the *Einsatzgruppen* (special operation squads) during the German invasion of the Soviet Union.

The mass murder of the Jews – the initial implementation of the so-called "Final Solution of the Jewish Problem" – was the fruit of a lengthy process: the gradual, widespread acceptance over decades, by the political community in Germany, of racial theory and its accompanying anti-Semitism. This culminated in the final confirmation by the Wannsee Conference on January 1942. Why and how racial theory and anti-Semitism became so influential, particularly among German physicians and medical students, is one of the questions which this book examines.

Sources of mutual attraction between Nazism and German physicians

The Canadian scholar, Michael Kater, noted that 44% of the German medical professionals were members of the Nazi Party. This was more than for any other academically trained profession. Among secondary-school teachers, in comparison, less than 15% were enlisted Party members. Moreover, 7% of the physicians were also members of the SS, the Nazi Party's black-uniformed special elite force.

Many of the German physicians hastened to join the Nazi Party only with its ascent to power. On the other hand, the Nazi student organizations had clear hegemony among German medical students well before the appointment of Hitler as Chancellor. The majority of medical students joined Nazi organizations at some time during their studies.

The profound involvement of German physicians and medical students with Nazism was, in many cases, opportunistic; many hoped to inherit the positions of their displaced Jewish colleagues. Before the Nazi rise to power, of a total 52,000 German physicians, some 8,500 (almost one in six) were Jews. Jewish physicians reached numbers far higher than the proportion of Jews in the general population. Prior to World War I, however, Jews had found it very difficult to establish themselves in the academic world, and rarely rose above the rank of *Privatdozent* – a low-salaried, nontenured lecturer. Non-Jewish colleagues made efforts to hamper Jewish entry to prestigious, specialist fields such as surgery or cardiology. Nevertheless, in certain unpopular specialties, such as dermatology, Jews represented over a third of all practitioners, and in the big cities such as Berlin, the proportion of physicians of Jewish descent was some 30%. Hospitals and health clinics made extensive use of their skills. In the interwar period, their numbers increased sharply among physicians acting in the service of federal states such as Prussia and Saxony, in municipalities and in schools. These positions were most desired by young German physicians.

Aside from opportunistic motives, it is clear that Nazi ideology was also of importance for a great number of German medical personnel who felt a genuine identification with the declared Nazi goals.

The secret of the appeal of Nazi ideology to physicians, and in particular to the younger ones among them, was its bio-racial vision – an essential part of Nazism. The very basis of Nazi ideology was a biological conception: the idea that the races of mankind are as separate and distinct as different species in the animal or plant kingdom, some being superior to others – with each race having its inherent physical characteristics, as well as its specific, inherited mental traits. Just as in Nature there are strong and weak creatures, and the strong win in the struggle for survival – so also with human races. The strong race, with its superior attributes, is designed by Nature to dominate those more inferior. Furthermore, since the Master Race is determined by its biological heredity, it must be kept pure, safe from being polluted and diluted by the blood of lesser races and defective individuals within itself. Such pollution and dilution would weaken the chances of survival of the race and obstruct the fulfillment of its historic destiny. As such, it was deemed the duty of those trained in biology, and especially of physicians, to be the guardians of racial purity.

Thus, according to Nazi thought, the physician not only contents himself with the traditional aims of Western medical tradition, the private treatment of the single patient towards his cure and recovery – that is, from an individual viewpoint. Instead, the teachers of the new doctrine maintained it should be incumbent upon the German physician to be, above all, the healer of the entire German people and to consider, first and foremost, the dictates of the German common national benefit as a whole and the fitness of its future generations. This new, necessary point of view should be collective rather than individual. The new task of the physician was to become a key functionary, a sort of gatekeeper, one meant to ensure that "unwanted" elements – whether from a racial aspect (first of all Jews, but also Gypsies and even Slavs) or from a genetic aspect (those afflicted with severe hereditary diseases) – would be kept out, and be prevented from contaminating the "community" of the German people (*Volksgemeinschaft*).

This lofty mission undoubtedly flattered the sense of importance of many physicians, making it easier for them to depart from accepted norms of Western medicine. From this point, there was but one step towards the sterilization and even extermination of those considered unfit and "unworthy" of life (*Lebensunwertig*). Some of the latter were even treated as human guinea pigs for medical experimentation in which physicians could be engaged free of any ethical restrictions. This would prove, in time, a considerable temptation for some SS doctors.

According to racial doctrine, race and genetics shared a common basis. Human racial difference is genetically determined, making some races "of inferior value" in the final analysis. German scholar Benno Müller-Hill expressed this view with succinct irony: "Jews are Jews and mentally-ill are mentally-ill because of their genes." Jews, psychiatric patients and other elements (dubbed "asocials" in Nazi terminology) were *a priori* "of inferior value" according to Nazi doctrine – in contrast with the healthy members of the full-blooded German *Volk*, those "of superior value." There was, therefore, no justification for the equality of the law for these two categories. They should be kept formally separate (as was accomplished through the law for sterilization and the Nuremberg Laws). It was important also to strive actively to increase the prominence of the "superior" elements over the "inferior" ones. Further, if it were proper to maintain such a "corrective discrimination" within Germany itself, it would seem fully justified to deal harshly when the time comes with less desirable elements – Slavs, for example – who could threaten the German superiority in the planned program of expansion eastwards which Hitler had promulgated in his **Mein Kampf**. The war of conquest for "living space" in the east, which he considered inevitable, seemed to him an opportune time to settle accounts with the "inferior" races.

Racial Theory

The roots of these concepts are easily found in the racial theories of the nineteenth century, and their supposed scientific fulfillment was the study of "Racial Hygiene" and Eugenics.

Throughout history, attempts have been made to find principles and rules for the classification of the human race. The differing skin color of peoples of various continents and regions served as a convenient point of departure for many thinkers, but also gave rise to many prejudices.

The Swedish father of taxonomy, Carl von Linné (Carolus Linnaeus), in his work **Systema Naturae** (1735) compared the various human races. He tried to define for each race distinct traits of personality, such as characterizing the Black race as lazy, superstitious and dissolute. From the middle of the nineteenth century, a more careful approach among scientists, especially anthropologists, was evident. They generally avoided fixing hierarchies to different racial groups. In this, they followed Charles Darwin, who usually avoided making value judgments about the nature of various groups of human origin, in contrast to the general nature of his theory of evolution; instead he emphasized the struggle for survival and the natural preference for improved species in the animal and vegetable world. His disciples were less careful. Scholars like the Briton, Herbert Spencer, who applied Darwinism to the social sphere, made it possible to develop trends of thought expounding the different value of various social groups from various origins. This trend of thought indirectly enabled economic liberalism and capitalism to flourish – by justifying the success of the "fittest" – and even justified colonialism, by talking about "the White Man's mission." The noted German biologist, Ernst Haeckel, developed Darwinist thought in Germany, and is attributed with the dubious equation "Darwinism = Selection." From his voluminous writings, the Nazis latched onto his notion that all aspects of life are underlain by biology – even politics, ethics and economics. They frequently quoted his statement that "politics is applied biology." The bitter fruit of such a conception reached its final ripening in Auschwitz.

The more sober-minded anthropologists were aware that, throughout history, there has been a constant interbreeding of races, particularly in Europe. This observation has been affirmed in our times, through advances in the study of genetics and DNA. It is now realized that there are no really, totally pure races – and the Jews are no exception. Environmental and climatic effects have no less an influence on human diversity than genetic causes.

In the nineteenth century, the subject of race achieved an enormous resonance with both the scientific community and the public, particularly in Germany. One possible reason for this was the country's political disunity. Unlike other European nations, Germany was not one unified sovereign state, with clearly defined borders, but was divided into many local authorities. The people did, however, harbor a sense of belonging culturally and ethnically to a German People (*Volk*). The mystique of race had a non-rational, romantic appeal, which complemented the myths cultivated by the proponents of German nationalism, in order to justify political union. Examples of such myths are the operas of Richard Wagner, glorifying the heritage of Teutonic mythology and the Germanic past. The anti-Semitism in his writings rounded out the circle.

However, advocates of the racial theories were not by necessity anti-Semitic, nor were they always German. Indeed, it was a Frenchman – Arthur de Gobineau – who created the "Aryan" myth of a white Master Race, in a peculiar blending of linguistic theories and aristocratic notions. In his well-known book, **An Essay on the Inequality of Human Races** (1855), he does not turn against the Jews. He viewed Palestine as a poor corner of the ancient world where the Jews of biblical time had proved the strength of a "high value" race in triumphing over the material conditions of their environment. He characterized the Jews as "a free, strong and intelligent nation of farmers and warriors, who have given rise to many learned and cultured individuals."

Gobineau regarded most of the White Race as the "Aryans," superior to the Yellow race he despised and the Black race he held in contempt. He was one of the first to warn of the supposed decline of the White Race through genetic degeneration and contamination caused by miscegenation with inferior races. In his last years, Gobineau befriended Cosima Wagner, the composer's widow. One of her friends translated his works into German, and so his ideas became current in right-wing German circles, such as the Pan-German League, which had a membership composed mostly of teachers. Some among them even omitted the words praising the Jews. The Orientalist, Lapogue, Gobineau's disciple, revised his teachings further, turning the Jews into the absolute enemy of the Aryan race.

Most influential in this field was Houston Stewart Chamberlain. Born the son of an English naval officer in 1855, Chamberlain was educated in Europe and made Germany his spiritual homeland. He became one of Wagner's slavish admirers, married his daughter Eva and made his home in Bayreuth, site of the yearly Wagner festivals. In his widely-read book, **The Foundations of the Nineteenth Century** (1899), Chamberlain glorified the Germans as standing at the helm of the Aryan and Nordic nations, representing the Jews on the opposite side, as their total antithesis and the very incarnations of Satan. This dichotomy became the fundamental basis of Nazi doctrine. He accepted as truisms all the anti-Semitic slanders, including **The Protocols of the Elders of Zion,** that notorious Russian forgery which appeared in print at the time. In his claim that race rules history, Chamberlain viewed the past as an everlasting conflict between Aryans and Semites.

Despite his description of the Germans as the real Chosen People, Chamberlain understood the difficulty of insisting on a uniform Nordic physical appearance for all Germans – tall, blond and blue-eyed – as it was obvious to any objective observer that this was far from the reality. With all his belief in the "Aryan type" and racism, he emphasized the character traits of the Germans as being decent, faithful and diligent, attributing to them a primordial Germanic Christianity, all of which formed what he called their specific "race spirit." He saw them as people still retaining their original superior Aryan characteristics. In contrast, he saw Jews as a mongrel riff-raff, descendents of ancient inferior races such as the Amorites and Hittites. In his view, the Jewish soul is materialistic, legalistic, quibbling, and lacking in tolerance and morality. He tried to prove his arguments by citing the Bible and the Talmud.

Chamberlain lived until 1927, aiding the Germans in their conflict in World War I against his native England. Shortly before he died he met Hitler, was deeply impressed by him and saw in him the future leader of Germany and of Europe. Hitler, in turn, was most influenced by Chamberlain's book, and regarded him as the harbinger of the Third Reich.

"Racial Hygiene" and Eugenics

From the beginning of the twentieth century, two complementary schools of thought, race hygiene and eugenics, flourished in Germany, seeking to achieve for themselves some measure of scientific respectability. The driving force behind these schools of thought was a sincere anxiety about the effects of degeneration (*Entartung*) and of hereditary diseases, current in Germany and other Western societies. Among the diseases provoking this anxiety were severe mental disorders such as schizophrenia, which were still incurable in spite of significant advances in their diagnosis and methods of treatment.

The study of "Racial Hygiene," initiated by Alfred Ploetz (who coined the term *Rassenhygiene* in 1895) and Wilhelm Schallmayer, strove to continue the work of past anthropologists with a detailed description of the differences between races by means of parameters such as physiognomic characteristics (eye shape and color, lip thickness and so forth), exacting skull measurements and comparison of other skeletal features.

The discovery of human blood types by Karl Landsteiner in 1900 strengthened the hope of proponents of Racial Hygiene that they would be able to base their researches on sound empirical findings. Racial Hygiene organizations flourished; the German Society for Racial Hygiene was established in 1904, its founders included senior government members, and it published an influential periodical. Even some Jews – Ignaz Zollschan best known among them – were members for a while, until they could no longer tolerate the anti-Semitic tendencies which began to permeate the Society.

After World War I, some of the most prominent racial hygienists, such as Eugen Fischer, Erwin Baur and Fritz Lenz rose to fame. They managed to be appointed as research directors of the Kaiser Wilhelm Society and were holders of university posts. Their writings were widely read. Their most important book, **Outline of Human Genetics and Racial Hygiene**, its first German edition[2] appearing in 1921, influenced Hitler very deeply. He read it while he was imprisoned after his failed

---

2   **Grundriß der menschlichen Erblichkeitslehre und Rassenhygiene.** München: Lehmann, 1921.

attempt to overthrow the government and seize the leadership of Germany in the Munich *Putsch* of 1923. In prison, Hitler dictated **Mein Kampf** to Rudolf Hess, copying into his manuscript several paragraphs from the book without taking excessive care about the accuracy of his quotations. His aim was to use – or in actuality to distort – a decent scientific publication (which did not employ anti-Semitic statements in its first edition) in order to further his own aims.

The word "hygiene" in the term "racial hygiene" hints at the practical and even preventive side of these teachings. Alfred Ploetz counted among the aims of the movement to campaign against the "two-children pattern" (desirably a boy and a girl) at the time considered ideal for a German family. The racial hygienists argued German families of good breeding should have more than two children in order to maintain the numerical balance of the Germans against their potential enemies. The goal was a balance of a race "of superior value" against the Russians and Poles of the Slavic race, whom they considered "of inferior value."

The German eugenic school, beginning in the last decade of the nineteenth century, was most explicit in its practical expression. Its name, Eugenics (from the Greek ευγενής: of good origin), declares its aims – the bearing of healthy offspring by worthy parents "of superior value," in order to perpetuate the future generations of suitable children (and soldiers) for the Homeland.

The proponents of eugenics argued the need for "constant maintenance" of the race: the prevention of marriage between those "of superior value" with partners carrying an unwanted genetic or racial heredity. It is possible to detect in these arguments the roots of the racist Nuremberg Laws of 1935, defending "the purity of German blood" against the Jews. But in the Weimar Republic (between the wars), the emphasis was as yet on the prevention of possible genetic defects among couples intending to marry. A network of marital consultation bureaus was established, for example in Berlin, the use of which was voluntary. In the twenties, such experts were limited to dispensing advice and using their powers of persuasion (though sometimes they gave an unequivocal recommendation not to marry or not to bear children). In the Nazi period, on the other hand, such consultation and advice became mandatory, and couples were not permitted to marry without being issued clearance from the eugenic experts.

Prior to the Nazi era, draconian measures such as sterilization and extermination (or "negative eugenics") were not seriously considered. The focus was on "Positive Eugenics"– encouraging procreation among those "of superior value" by means of financial incentives, such as easy mortgages for housing, and discouraging those "of inferior value," for example through taxation. Similar means were occasionally used against those "of superior value" who refused to bear children, such as unmarried elderly singles, homosexuals, and married couples who declined to have children.

Already in his programmatic book, Hitler had stated very explicitly that a decent German must not bring children into the world if he was not sure that they would enjoy good health. The meaning of his words became all too clear once he held power. In July 1933 the Nazis passed a law enabling forced sterilization of those suffering from hereditary diseases. By this act, the ethical boundary was crossed from the acceptance of the basic human rights of the individual in Western democracies to spurning these rights in the name of the national collective. Thus, on rising to power, the Nazis quickly transformed the ideas of racial hygiene into absolute laws, and charged the physicians of Germany with the responsibility for their implementation.

Further reading

Michael H. Kater. **Doctors under Hitler.** Chapel Hill: University of North Carolina Press, 1989 [A German edition appeared in 2000].

Hans-Walter Schmuhl. **Rassenhygiene, Nationalsozialismus, Euthanasie; Von der Verhütung zur Vernichtung "lebensunwerten Lebens," 1890-1945.** Göttingen: Vandenhoeck & Ruprecht, 1987.

Paul Weindling. **Health, Race, and German Politics between National Unification and Nazism, 1870-1945.** Cambridge: Cambridge University Press, 1989.

Sheila F. Weiss. **Race Hygiene and National Efficiency: The Eugenics of Wilhelm Schallmeyer.** Berkeley: University of California Press, 1987.

Chapter 2

Sterilization in Nazi Germany

One of the first laws to reflect the spirit of the new Nazi rulers of Germany was the law requiring the sterilization of humans euphemistically termed the Law for Prevention of Hereditary-Ill (*erbkranken*) Offspring. It was passed by the Reichstag on July 14, 1933, and put into effect at the beginning of 1934. The date of the Reichstag vote – Bastille Day – was not chosen by accident. The new rulers desired to put aside the ethical heritage of Human Rights inherited from the French Revolution, and in its place emphasize the different and unequal racial and genetic worth of the various segments of the German population. Germany, however, was not the only state where sterilization of men and women had been preached and practiced, nor was it the first. In effect, many countries have had legalized sterilization for eugenic reasons including India, China, Canada, the United States and a number of Scandinavian and South American countries.

The school of Eugenics in the West

The notion of preventing those births unwanted from an eugenic point of view, which involved clear principles of racial hygiene, had been current in some fundamentally democratic states even prior to the twentieth century. Ideas of betterment and preservation of the race (with reference almost exclusively to Caucasians) had been gaining attention since the rise of the theories of racial hygiene and of social Darwinism. Many scientists were concerned about the perceived threats confronting the dominant classes in developed countries, such as Germany. Much was made of the threat of social degradation and biological degeneration posed by the rapid proliferation of socially marginal elements. These elements were considered to be lacking the moral restraints attributed to the more educated and affluent strata of society. Concern about the rapid population increase of the Chinese and Japanese ("the Yellow Peril"), potentially challenging the world hegemony of the White race in the heyday of White colonial imperialism, was always in the background of these worries.

An additional source of concern was the large influx of immigrants from Eastern Europe, including many Jews, some of whom chose to remain in Central Europe, although the desired goal of most was emigration to the United States. Much anxiety was expressed over the possible upsurge in crime that this might cause. Many feared the immigrants as potential carriers of hereditary diseases, which were difficult to discern and screen out in the perfunctory examinations carried out in immigration centers like Ellis Island, at the entrance to New York Harbor.

Even though immigration quotas set by the government had a somewhat limiting effect, American pioneers of the Eugenic School, such as Charles Davenport and Harry Laughlin, had been arguing for even stricter controls for the waves of immigration. Their influence became evident in the more stringent Immigration Act of 1924. Additionally, they advocated extending the legislation in America for sterilization, which had been in operation in several states from the beginning of the twentieth century. In those states, young people of both sexes, many of them immigrant children who were thought to be carriers of genetic illnesses, underwent sterilization. While most states did not allow sterilization, some were more permissive in this regard. The formal and surgical procedures required, in every case, the consent of the patient or his legal guardian. Many of the patients, generally adolescents reaching sexual maturity, suffered from various degrees of mental retardation or illness. The majority of such hospitalized cases were schizophrenic patients, most of whom, since the onset of their condition generally appeared in their early twenties, were adults.

Some of those sterilized in the United States were not suffering from hereditary illnesses at all, but were simply inmates of institutions for children and adolescents from broken or destitute families. The Virginia State Colony for Epileptics and Feebleminded at Lynchburg, an institute founded to treat and take care of such children, became infamous for carrying out thousands of sterilizations, the majority of which lacked any medical justification.

The sterilization of males was generally performed by vasectomy. The brutal method of castration was mainly reserved for sex offenders, in order to suppress their sexual drive, in addition to rendering them infertile. In some cases, the vasectomy was later reversible, with the reconnection of the *vas deferens*. For females, however, the procedure was more complicated: from total hysterectomy to salpingectomy or tubal ligation, and was fraught with greater danger, required hospitalization, and involved the risk of complication and even death.

In 1922 Harry Laughlin proposed a "Model Eugenical Sterilization Law," based on the experience in those states that had adopted varying sterilization legislation. He argued an ostensibly modern idea – that the sterilization of mentally disabled and non-violent psychiatric patients would free them from confinement in institutions, enabling their freedom of movement within the community at large. They could have useful contact with other people without the risk of their being able to bear children who could become a burden for them and for society in general.

This mixture of eugenic arguments claiming benefits for the entire society – saving the expense of institutionalizing patients, and claims for the good of the victims themselves – all fostered agitation for sterilization in America.

Later, in Nazi Germany, very similar arguments were used to justify medically sanctioned murder, euphemistically termed "Euthanasia."

According to statistics compiled from the fourteen American states where sterilization had been practiced (with California in the lead), the total number of sterilizations from 1900 to 1933 amounted to somewhat less than 27,000, averaging 800 a year. This figure is definitely low, in comparison to the unprecedented high number of sterilized persons in Nazi Germany.

The policy of sterilization in Nazi Germany

From 1934 to the outbreak of World War II – less than six years – about 380,000 men and women were sterilized in Nazi Germany.[1] In the first

---

1   The exact figures were never officially disclosed in Nazi Germany. The number
     mentioned reflects a certain compromise between different estimates (such as those
     of Gerhard Baader and Gisela Bock).

year of the implementation of the sterilization law in Germany, more people were sterilized than in an entire generation in the United States. Alfons Labisch drew our attention in his research to a law of vital importance, which was enacted in July 1934, a year after the sterilization law.[2] This law – "Unifying the health services" – enabled to implement on grand scale the sterilization law in the municipalities as well as the rural areas. The newly appointed Nazi doctors in the provincial Health Offices *(Gesundheitsämter)* wished to prove their adherence to the recently defined "population policy" by active pursuit of the "inferior" people and recommended to sterilize many of them.

The number of sterilizations reflected Nazi thoroughness and a determination by the authorities to accomplish the declared goals of eugenics. In this, they provoked the envy of devotees of eugenic theories the world over.

The sterilization legislation reflected the stubborn determination of several German psychiatrists and medical practitioners to "purify" the German people from what they considered to be the encumbering burden of "unfit" elements: patients with severe mental illnesses thought to have a genetic basis, congenital feebleminded, and other inherited gross disabilities. Ernst Rüdin (1874-1952) was the first and foremost of those seeking a practical solution. He had studied under Emil Kraeplin, one of the pioneer researchers of schizophrenia at the beginning of the twentieth century. Kraeplin was, essentially, the first to describe in detail the symptoms and progress of the disease. Rüdin's own studies led him to believe that genetics were the chief cause of the illness, a far-reaching pronouncement which lacked a firm statistical validity. Ernst Rüdin and others thus persevered in trying to extend and verify the statistical and genealogical evidence for Kraeplin's assertion, of the absolute aeteological dominance of the genetic factor, which few doubted.

Rüdin was one of the founders of the Berlin branch of the German Society for Race Hygiene (1905), which had as a mission, among other things, advancing research on the family genetics of those deemed "of inferior value," and preventing the reproduction of patients suffering

2   A. Labisch / Florian Tennstedt: **Der Weg zum "Gesetz über die Vereinheitlichung Des Gesundheitswesens", vom 3. Juli 1934.** Düsseldorf: Akademie für Öffentliches Gesundheitswesen, 1985.

from hereditary diseases. Rüdin's advancement as professor of psychiatry in Munich and Basel aided his appointment to key positions in the Kaiser Wilhelm Institute. In 1932, on the eve of the Nazi rise to power, he was chosen to become president of the Society for Race Hygiene and helped the Nazis in granting a respectable scientific aura to some of their designs in the realm of "race improvement." He composed commentaries on the sterilization law, including detailed instructions for its implementation. About ten years after the passage of the law, for which he was instrumental in drafting, lobbying and justifying, Rüdin praised the Nazi regime, saying: "only through [Hitler's] work has our thirty-year-long dream of translating race hygiene into action finally become a reality."

Rüdin served the Nazis as the Reich's Commissioner for Race Hygiene. By means of the voluminous amount of data he had accumulated for years, he sought to prove the connection between heredity and many illnesses. A large part of this data was included in the sterilization law. Much of his research was devoted to investigating what he considered to be the strong linkage of hereditary diseases with crime and other "asocial" behaviors.

The physician, Arthur Gütt, who served at the time as a consultant in the Nazi Ministry of the Interior, and later on as one of its directors, and chairman of the Academy for Public Health, acknowledged that it would have been difficult to pass the sterilization law without Rüdin's prestige and renown.

The sterilization law and its implementation

This law was applicable to nine categories of candidates for sterilization:

- Congenital feebleminded (idiots and imbeciles)
- Schizophrenics
- Manic-depressives
- Congenital epileptics
- Cases of Huntington's chorea (a degenerative central nervous disease typified by involutional, purposeless motor movements and behavioral changes)
- Congenitally blind

- Congenitally deaf
- Congenitally physically deformed
- Heavy alcoholics.

Several of these categories seem dubious – and not only from a modern point of view. Being effectively treatable, epilepsy, for example, does not really constitute a debilitating disability. Even in Nazi Germany, some physicians had their doubts about several of these categories. The genetic component of alcoholism, for example, does not seem to carry any real weight. At most, the environmental factor may be attributable for its damaging influence on children. It is evident that Rüdin and his colleagues sought to extend the law to encompass all those they considered "asocial." Even with regard to illnesses having a less questionable hereditary basis, such as schizophrenia, doubts were voiced, since the condition is not generally transmitted directly from parents to children. Sometimes it may appear only after skipping a generation or two, emerging often only in more distant relatives, such as cousins.[3]

A survey was undertaken in 1934 of 106 directors of psychiatric institutions. Most respondents did not predict beneficial effects for their institutions from sterilization in the foreseeable future. Some of the directors commented that the difficulty of sterilizing schizophrenics in Germany would be truly considerable, since millions of Germans had family members who were schizophrenics – even if only distantly related. Even then, it would require a number of generations to elapse in order to know if the disease in Germany has indeed been eradicated. Clearly this was not feasible, if only for the reluctance of the Nazi leadership to allow the resulting, considerable demographic depletion of the German population.

German physicians were required to report all patients ill with hereditary diseases and fit for sterilization. The network of marital advice stations (the use of which for couples intending to marry had become compulsory) was an additional source of information for the authorities. The victims were usually selected for sterilization by physicians – officials of the regional health office (*Gesundheitsamt*) in towns or rural

---

3   **Medicine, Ethics, and the Third Reich** (Edited by John J. Michalczyk). Kansas City, Missouri: Sheed & Ward, 1994, p. 44 [D. Nadav].

areas. These were nearly always Nazi Party members, the Jews and left-wing elements having been weeded out. The officials ordered the victims to report to a nearby hospital for the surgical procedure. If they refused, the police would forcibly escort them despite their objections.

The Nazis made an attempt to preserve an ostensible appearance of formal adherence to the law and to blur its compulsory nature. A special nation-wide network of Heredity Courts was established for this purpose, each composed of three members: a lawyer as chairman and two physicians. Here, too, at least two of the members were always Nazis. Appearing before these courts, victims were granted the right to appeal the decision to sterilize them – but such appeals usually failed. In a very few cases – less than a tenth – their appeal was upheld. The decisions were often based on perfunctory evidence. People presumed to be of limited intelligence were asked supposedly common-knowledge questions, such as "Who was Bismarck?" When on one occasion, a rural woman answered, "a herring," her unexpected response occasioned some learned deliberation, and her reply was deemed acceptable. That great statesman had indeed been an avid consumer of pickled herring marinated in salt and vinegar, of a type that was subsequently named "Bismarck" in his honor.

Even after they won their appeal, the appellants' personal medical details were recorded on special heredity cards. Further, by the late thirties, a central registry of all these cases was in the planning. Under this plan, later partially effected, all sterilized victims, as well as other suspected persons, were to be listed on this card registry. A special category was a list of tens of thousands of Gypsies also considered "of inferior value." With the introduction of the forerunner of computers, the authorities began to compile the information on perforated cards produced by the American firm, Hollerith. By these means, the Nazi totalitarian dictatorship wished to assure itself control and immediate access to eugenic information, enabling further reviews, and even medical murder, for those deemed to be suffering from real or imagined disabilities.

Surgical sterilizations resulted in hundreds of lives lost, mainly women, for whom the procedure was considerably more complicated. The fatalities, presaging the Nazis' full Euthanasia Program, were never revealed at the time to the German public.

German propagandists recognized extensive, systematic action was needed to prepare the ground for further sterilization actions, and for the more severe measures already being planned. From the mid-thirties, propaganda posters were published graphically emphasizing the heavy economic burden imposed on the German people by having to support a vast number of "freeloaders." One such poster exhibited a sturdy German worker carrying on his shoulders two misshapen figures. The inscription noted that the economic cost to the German taxpayers to institutionalize and care for two such chronic patients cost as much as supporting, with ease, four upstanding working families. Other posters alleged a vastly disproportionate reproduction rate among the hereditarily diseased and "asocials" in comparison with the normal birth rate of the "healthy" German population.

Considerations of racial hygiene without even the most tenuous justification of preventing hereditary illnesses also occurred. Only in 1979 was it revealed that in 1937 the Gestapo, in Cologne and a number of other cities, had carried out a program of enforced sterilization for several hundred young people of mixed parentage – even through the victims were free of any hereditary disease or defect.[4] Those affected, born about a dozen years previously, were the children of German women and dark-skinned soldiers mostly from Morocco and Senegal. These soldiers were serving in the French expeditionary forces in the Rhineland, whose presence was designed to assure the payment of the heavy indemnities forced upon Germany by the Treaty of Versailles. These offspring, derogatorily referred to as "Rhineland Bastards," were considered "inferior" and totally unwanted according to Nazi racial standards. To prevent them from passing their supposedly "inferior" genes onto the next generation, they were compulsorily sterilized upon reaching puberty.

With the outbreak of war, the campaign for sterilization was stopped. These measures had become redundant, with the decision to simply put these helpless victims to death by means of medical methods and the use of subterfuge. In this, the Nazis relied fully, as before, on the collaboration of unscrupulous German medical personnel.

---

4   Reiner Pommerin. **"Sterilisierung der Rheinlandbastarde"; Das Schicksal einer farbigen deutschen Minderheit 1918-1937.** Düsseldorf: Droste, 1979.

Further reading

Gisela Bock. **Zwangssterilisation im Nationalsozialismus; Studien zur Rassenpolitik und Frauenpolitik.** Opladen: Westdeutscher Verlag, 1986.

Deadly Medicine; Creating the Master Race [US Holocaust Memorial Museum]. Chapel Hill, N.C.: University of North Carolina Press, 2004. Ch. 4 (written by Gisela Bock).

Robert Proctor. **Racial Hygiene: Medicine under the Nazis.** Cambridge, Mass.: Harvard University Press, 1988.

Chapter 3

Proper Medicine in Nazi Germany: A Paradox?

German medicine and natural science were widely esteemed in the beginning of the twentieth century. German medical research was regarded as being at the very forefront of world scientific advances. German physicians often served as pioneers in developing techniques which gained application only in the following generation. Such was the case, in 1929, of Werner Forssmann, the pioneer of cardiac catheterization, who performed this procedure for the first time ever on himself at the provincial hospital in Eberswalde. His innovation was overlooked until it was rediscovered by American scientists after World War II.

In the first decades of the century, the number of German nationals among Nobel Prize winners was remarkable (a considerable portion of them Jews). Robert Koch, Albert Neisser, and Paul Ehrlich – the latter two Germans of Jewish descent – earned universal acclaim for their discovery of the causes of, and cures for, tuberculosis, cholera, anthrax, gonorrhea and syphilis, together with proposing the theory of chemotherapy. German scientists were responsible for important discoveries, such as the EEG (electroencephalograph), X-rays, and even Aspirin, the work mainly of the Jewish-born chemist, Arthur Eichengrün.

German universities were remarkable for their high levels of scholarship. The United States had not yet attained leadership in the field of medical research. Outstanding students from many countries showed a particular preference for rounding off their medical training at renowned German universities, such as Heidelberg and Berlin. The German scientific community accorded prestige to physicians engaged in research and experimentation, and the drive to publish and to innovate was a constant motivation for many of them.

During the Nazi period, this tradition of reverence for medical experimentation and research still continued – but with little regard for the ethical questions involved. A few German scientists won Nobel prizes even in that period, Adolf Butenhandt, for example, who received in 1939 the prize for his work on the hormones responsible for human sexual identity. In those years, Germany indeed continued to maintain its high standing in medicine – provided that the patients did not belong to one of the groups considered by the regime to be of inferior value: ranging from Jews and Gypsies to individuals afflicted with certain hereditary illnesses, whether actual or imagined.

The sound medical practice that existed in Nazi Germany was not immune to the Nazi doctrine of racial hygiene. An example of this was the sterilization of the Afro-Germans in 1937, a deed, which transgressed the boundaries of what flimsy legitimacy the Nazis strove to attribute to themselves in the first years of their regime. Even homosexuals were regarded as showing tendencies endangering the German people ("asocial" in Nazi parlance, together with beggars and idlers) – and not a few of them were persecuted and dispatched to concentration camps.

Many German research institutes continued to be active during the Nazi era, being supported in the thirties by the American Rockefeller Foundation and other prestigious institutes. Some were assisted, of course, by well-known German bodies such as the *Deutsche Forschungsgemeinschaft* (DFG, the German Research Community). Not all of these institutions engaged, in the thirties, in the dubious issues of racial doctrine. Later on, however, they also began aiding in unethical medical undertakings, such as some of the "experiments" conducted in Auschwitz. These findings came to light only a generation after the War. The contemporary German geneticist, Benno Müller-Hill, played a central role in exposing such facts, while examining in the 1980s the deeds of his colleagues and teachers during the Nazi period.[1]

Despite this, however, the foundations of German medical practice and scholarship had been sound enough prior to Nazi ascendancy to influence the medical sector during the dozen years of Nazi dictatorship

---

1   Benno Müller-Hill. **Murderous Science.** Oxford: Oxford University Press, 1988 [the original German edition appeared in 1984 as was mentioned before].

as well. Much of the research conducted in Germany in the late thirties and early forties is still considered of importance.

Cancer research in Nazi Germany

A surprising fact which has only been made publicly known a decade ago was that the connection between smoking and lung cancer and other diseases was first discovered and studied in Nazi Germany. It was likewise the first country to initiate a public campaign against smoking and its dangers. This campaign was launched by means of posters, radio broadcasts and propaganda films, predating by one generation the similar efforts made in this direction in the United States starting in the sixties.

The anti-smoking campaign in Germany went beyond the declarative level: an active effort was made towards the early diagnosis of diseases such as cancer of the lung and the breast, and mass examinations of those likely to be at risk were carried out, as is customary today. Diagnostic instruments were designed – such as the colposcope (invented by Hans Hinselmann), making the early discovery of cervical cancer in women easier. Questionable experiments were conducted in Auschwitz to test the efficacy of the colposcope on women suspected of being cancer-prone. In such cases, their entire wombs were often brutally excised and sent for examination.

An American scholar, Robert Proctor, who cannot be suspected of sympathy towards Nazis, and who even published an important study of the criminal implications of racial hygiene,[2] has written a book titled **The Nazi War on Cancer.** This book shows that though many Jewish cancer researchers like Hans Sachs were dismissed from their posts[3] – as were other Jewish scientists in many fields – cancer research was not hampered too significantly. The famous Nobel-prize winning scientist, Otto Warburg, a half-Jew, was even permitted to continue directing the Kaiser Wilhelm Institute of Cell Physiology during the entire Nazi

---

2   **Racial Hygiene: Medicine under the Nazis.** Cambridge, Mass.: Harvard University Press, 1988.

3   A useful list appeared at the time: **List of Displaced German Scholars.** London: Notgemeinschaft Deutscher Wissenschaftler im Ausland, 1936. Prof. Sachs is mentioned on p. 58.

period. He was certainly aided in this by his ties with the Rockefeller Foundation. Even Hitler's close associates in his private office, Philip Bouhler and Viktor Brack, saw fit to allow Warburg to continue in his post "for the benefit of the world" – as they claimed after the War. They also believed (erroneously) that he knew the solution to the riddle of cancer and its treatment.

Undoubtedly, Hitler, being a consistent non-smoker, influenced Nazi cancer studies. He and his close advisers granted their full support to studies focused on smoking evidenced by massive financial grants to researchers. Accordingly, a special institute – the first in the world – to study the harmful effects of smoking was founded in 1941 in Jena, its funding granted directly from Hitler's office. SS physician Karl Astel, one of Himmler's protegés, was appointed as its director. Robert Proctor tells us that two of the scientists employed in it, Schairer and Schoeniger, published in 1943 a sizeable statistical survey based on the analysis of five previous studies, providing final confirmation of the correlation between smoking and cancer, as well as additional afflictions such as heart disease.

The Nazi campaign against smoking, however, was not free of non-medical considerations. The anti-Semitic prejudice of Hitler and Nazi ideology was evident here as well. Tobacco manufacturers were represented as Jewish capitalists enjoying enormous profits from the sales of a toxic product. This underscored the oft-heard theme of the virulent, anti-Semitic propaganda of the time – the representation of the Jews as a cancer spreading throughout the body of the German nation.

By the beginning of 1939, Aryan cigarette manufacturers, such as Philip Reemtsma, were already protesting against being represented in the public eye as spreading harmful substances. Nonetheless, according to Proctor, they announced their readiness to lower the levels of nicotine in their products.

The school of "New German Medicine"

Hitler's influence was evident also in another sphere of health policy. The Führer, as is well-known, was an avowed vegetarian, and showed interest in fostering theories of natural healing based upon the use of herbal remedies and a holistic approach. Homeopathy, with its deep roots in German folk medicine, also among these theories, together constituted what was known for some years as "The New German School of Healing." Heinrich Himmler, Head of the SS, and Rudolf Hess, Hitler's deputy, were greatly interested in these practices. A hospital named after Hess, specializing in "natural" curing methods, was established in Dresden, long known for its alternative healing centers and a world famous Hygiene Museum.[4] Himmler for his part encouraged the followers of this new school of medical practice and supported them within his own realm of authority – the SS and the concentration camps, in which various plants for the purpose of medical experimentation were cultivated. Dachau concentration camp in particular became famous for its extensive fields of medicinal herbs. German priests accused of opposition activities were employed in this work. Some of the physicians under Himmler's patronage, like Adolf Pokorny and Carl Clauberg, used these fields to grow herbs for their experimental work. Pokorny believed that the resin of a South American plant, *Caladium seguinium*, could be useful in preventing pregnancy. He intended to employ this resin against Jewish and Slav women, so as to enable their use as slave laborers without the danger of their reproducing. This illustrates the potential evil and distorted use of seemingly innocuous findings. The experiments, however, were unsuccessful, as the plant could not thrive in the Dachau plantations.

"The New German School of Healing" would thus have been used to serve as an additional weapon in the planned biological elimination of "inferior" races. It is worth noting, however, that most German physicians were not enthusiastic about these new curative systems, which had gained a semi-official approval. The majority of German doctors practicing in the Nazi era had received their training in conventional medical methods (*Schulmedizin*), and thus were reluctant to substitute their previous knowledge with theories whose scientific

---

4   According to information kindly granted to me by Prof. C.P. Heidel, Dresden's museum played a part in spreading Nazi racist and eugenic propaganda in the thirties. Strangely enough some Jews had an important role in the spread of alternative medicine prior to the Nazi takeover. D. Nadav, "Julius Moses' Einstellung zur Kurierfreiheit," in: C.P. Heidel (Ed.), **Naturheilkunde und Judentum**. Frankfurt am Main: Mabuse-Verlag, 2008. pp. 163-170.

worth had not been sufficiently proven. An overt struggle between the two systems ensued, with clear economic imperatives at stake – the competition for patients. Eventually, conventional medicine gained the upper hand, especially after the demise in 1939 of Gerhard Wagner, the *"Führer"* of the NS Physicians' League and a devotee of the school of New German Medicine. Erwin Liek, a leading ideologue of the new direction, designated to become director of the Dresden hospital, had died in 1935. Rudolf Hess' flight to Britain in 1941, hoping to achieve peace with England, was seen by many as a betrayal and played a part in discrediting in the public eye the image of the "New German Medicine," with which Hess had been associated.

Medical studies

The dispute between the two schools of medical thought raises the question of the nature of regular medical training in German universities. Conventional medical studies during the Nazi period differed somewhat from those in the preceding era.[5] One obvious difference was, of course, the exclusion of Jewish lecturers and students from universities. Jewish instructors were promptly dismissed in 1933. In some cases, their military service during World War I was a mitigating factor, but with the death in 1934 of Field Marshal Hindenburg, the German President who had insisted upon these extenuating circumstances for his former colleagues-at-arms, this restraint was eliminated.

Among the students, the change was somewhat slower. Already-enrolled Jewish students were at first allowed to finish their studies, and new students were permitted to enroll, subjected to a severely restricted admission quota (*"numerus clausus"*). Even this state of affairs was not always maintained as the authorities turned a blind eye towards the violent behavior of Nazi students in many universities towards their Jewish fellows. Towards the end of the thirties, a sweeping ban on Jewish students in universities was enforced, in parallel with the revoking in July 1938 of all practice permits of Jewish medical personnel.

5   Hendrik van den Bussche. **Im Dienste der "Volksgemeinschaft" – Studienreform im Nationalsozialismus am Beispiel der ärztlichen Ausbildung.** Berlin und Hamburg: Reimer, 1989.

There were in general no radical changes in the contents of medical teaching in Nazi Germany, save for the introduction of ideologically tainted studies, which were added to the curriculum. These were, principally, courses in racial hygiene and human genetics from the Nazi standpoint. Scientific institutes dealing with these matters had already been established in the early twenties in various places across Germany, and now new university lecturers for these subjects, mostly Nazis, were appointed. Nine additional chairs of Race Studies were established during the Nazi period. Difficulty arose in the appointment of new professors. The relative scarcity of qualified people, who could prove by their appropriate publications that they were deserving of promotion, meant it was difficult to fill positions. In some medical schools, deans displayed courage and blocked the advance to professorship in these fields of undeserving candidates, despite the generous government subsidies offered to the schools and Nazi pressure.

Starting in 1936, with the increased size of the army and its preparation towards possible war, special courses dealing with the treatment of combat injuries were added. On the other hand, a gradual decrease was observed in the courses considered too theoretical and affected by what was derided as "Jewish over-intellectualism." This was accompanied by a tendency to shorten both the period of study and the lengthy internship characteristic of medical studies in Germany prior to the Nazi era.

Students and lecturers who joined the SS in masses were sent for additional training: a combination of lectures in the Nazi spirit with physical fitness training and military exercises. Special camps were established for this purpose, in scenic surroundings – generally near medieval castles – which were meant to remind the participants of the glory of medieval Germanic military orders. Whole classes of students and doctors were sent there, housed in dormitories by rotation. The most famous place of study for SS doctors was the castle Alt Rhese, on the banks of a picturesque lake in north Germany. Participation in such courses was not compulsory for ordinary medical practitioners, but served as a springboard for further advance to more valued positions.

During the war years, an accelerated effort to shorten the duration of study and pare down the curriculum was evident. With the war unabating, the German army (*Wehrmacht*) needed many medical servicemen, particularly on the eastern front. In Stalingrad alone some 600 doctors fell or were taken prisoner. Medical training was shortened in 1942 to a mere ten semesters. Following appeals to women, many female students entered medical schools as well, and on finishing their studies, were directed mainly to treat the civilian population, which suffered severe casualties in the increasingly heavier bombing of German cities. Half a million civilians were killed in these bombings, and millions more were wounded and were in need of some sort of medical care. Many hospitals were destroyed as well, and efforts were needed to provide makeshift medical services at a reasonable level. Furthermore, most of the seriously wounded soldiers were sent back to Germany from the front for continuing treatment. Some of them where housed in former Jewish hospitals (in Hamburg and Breslau, for example), confiscated from Jewish communities and whose patients and doctors had been sent to extermination camps. Elderly German physicians, no longer suitable for military duty, were employed in the care of the civilian wounded, toiling to exhaustion for twelve to fourteen hours a day.

In addition to the hardships within the hospitals, a shortage of medications developed as well. These – especially the new drugs, such as sulfa or antibiotics like penicillin, needed at the front – were meagerly portioned out to the civilian population. This gave rise to a black market for such medicines.

The collaboration of physicians with the Nazi regime

Perhaps the worst transgression of German physicians was the widespread breaking of established medical ethics in order to collaborate with the Nazis and implement their ideology. This phenomenon increasingly worsened as the Nazis became more established in power and broadened their measures against the "racially inferior," with ostensible medical excuses. German doctors betrayed the trust of their patients, people who depended on them to act in their best interests under all circumstances.

It appears that many German physicians were not at all troubled by the fact that their collaboration with the regime made a mockery of accepted moral values, including medical ethics. The discrimination against Jewish patients, for instance, while segregating their treatment from those of Aryan patients (in accordance with the Nuremberg Laws) was contrary to the Hippocratic Oath, which physicians were obliged to swear on the conclusion of their studies – an oath which was not rescinded even during the Nazi era.

German physicians generally appeared to have welcomed the discriminatory measures against their Jewish colleagues, benefiting from the eliminated competition. They were able to occupy the places and practices of the ousted Jewish practitioners, replacing them in public service and taking over their lists of patients. None of the German doctors ever publicly voiced protest over the persecution of their Jewish colleagues. At most, some of them helped their Jewish friends in secret by writing letters of recommendation upon their emigration from Germany.

Distinguished physicians, like the famous surgeon Ferdinand Sauerbruch, often hid behind the mask of political non-involvement, in order to justify their continuing collaboration with the Nazi authorities. True, Sauerbruch himself was not a supporter of the Nazi party, and even helped one of his former loyal assistants, the Jewish Prof. Rudolf Nissen, to find shelter and work in Turkey. In more subtle ways, however, he served the Nazi regime and even lent it a measure of prestige by accepting prizes and honors. Only a small minority of famous German practitioners left their country, in contrast to writers such as Thomas Mann and Bertolt Brecht.

A sizeable portion of the Jewish doctors, forced to emigrate from Germany, landed in Palestine, quadrupling the numbers of local physicians there within two years. In October 1935, the British Mandatory government in Palestine forbade the issue of new work permits for physicians to prevent the economic collapse of the medical profession. Judging historically, the German immigrants contributed decisively towards modernizing medical services within the Jewish community of Palestine and to Palestinian society at large.

Not infrequently, German doctors acted from an ideological impulse without any medical necessity, even causing damage to those under their care, in complete contradiction of the foremost demand of the Hippocratic Oath: *"Non nocere"* – Do no harm. In October 1937, Prof. Otmar von Verschuer, director of the Kaiser Wilhelm Institute of Anthropology, Human Heredity and Eugenics in Frankfurt, appealed to the German Minister of Justice, complaining that the court disregarded his opinion when accepting a defendant's petition not to be decreed a full-blooded Jew under the Nuremberg Laws, since his mother had had an Aryan lover before his birth. Verschuer and his assistant (Josef Mengele) based their opinion upon blood and tissue tests of all involved. They insisted that the father had really been a Jew, and did not take at all into consideration the harmful implications for the future of the person concerned.

Later on, and from an entirely different motive, SS doctors collaborated in the act of kidnapping children of Aryan appearance in occupied countries, mainly in Poland. Such children, mostly orphans, were brought to Germany and put in institutes belonging to the "Source of Life" (*Lebensborn*) network, under the aegis of the SS.[6] The children were raised as Germans, and SS doctors like Gregor Ebner took part in diagnosing them "fit for Germanization" and in taking care of them until their maturity.

The readiness on the part of German physicians to grant priority to political considerations, even though these were patently unprofessional, cleared the way for ever more drastic measures, beginning at first with the sterilization and the murder of helpless patients, and leading to genocide, directed chiefly against the Jewish people.

Further reading

Johanna Bleker and Norbert Jachertz (eds.). **Medizin im "Dritten Reich."** Köln: Deutscher Ärzte-Verlag, 1993 [2. ed.].

Fridolf Kudlien. **Ärzte im Nationalsozialismus.** Köln: Kiepenheuer & Witsch, 1985.

Robert Proctor. **The Nazi War on Cancer.** Princeton, N.J.: Princeton University Press, 1999.

Christian Pross and Götz Aly (eds.). **The Value of Man; Medicine in Germany 1918-1945.** Berlin, Edition Hentrich, 1989. A German edition: **Das Wert des Menschen; Medizin in Deutschland 1918-1945,** appeared simultaneously.

---

6   Georg Lilienthal. **Der "Lebensborn e. V.";Ein Instrument nationalsozialistischer Rassenpolitik.** München: Urban und Fischer, 1985 [Neue erw. Ausgabe: Fischer Taschenbuch, 2004].

Chapter 4
"Mercy Killing" (Euthanasia) in Nazi Germany

The gradual sanctioning in Germany, before the War, of what was euphemistically called euthanasia (mercy killing) was the prelude to full-scale genocide. Under this program, hundreds of thousands of Aryan Germans, whose only fault was their being afflicted with a severe disease, were deprived of their life under the pretext of "mercy killing."

The sterilization of the so-called "Rhineland Bastards" (as described in Chapter 2) breached the legal boundaries previously limiting sterilization – for example, the existence of Heredity Courts, which heard (at least in theory) appeals in cases of planned sterilization and were empowered to overrule the dire decrees. The sterilization of young people of "mixed" blood in 1937 was certainly a criminal act, devoid of any legal sanction. It was a clear case where racist considerations proved more powerful than any medical necessity. The next step on the slippery road downwards was inevitable – the killing of people suffering from gross defects.

Euthanasia since the Weimar Republic

The idea of euthanasia had been debated a number of years before under the democratic Weimar Republic. In 1920, psychiatrist Alfred Hoche and law professor Karl Binding published a book, the title of which left nothing to the imagination: **The Permission for the Elimination** [*Vernichtung*] **of the Life of the Unworthy of Living** [*lebensunwerten Lebens*]. The justification for such permission was simple: some individuals, mainly those seriously retarded from birth or severely mentally ill, whom they argued were "mentally or intellectually dead" and whose life lacked "a subjective and objective value" – especially those committed to institutions – constituted a heavy material burden on society. Because of the difficult economic conditions of Germany after its defeat in World War I, it was arguable to examine the possibility of aiding some of them, in particular the hopelessly incurable, to end their lives without pain and suffering. Both writers were careful in their wording, and some of their claims reflect the arguments that persist until today in favor of mercy killing for humanitarian reasons. Nonetheless, their book provoked a public outcry, and the subject was dropped. Dr. Boeters, a physician who openly expressed similar views, was dismissed from his official position.

With the improvement of the economic situation during the 1920s, the subject receded from the attention of most – except for Hitler and his followers, who took it up. Some of Hitler's conversations from these years are preserved, in which he talked about the liquidation of useless "freeloaders" as he called them – chronic patients and others of "inferior value" who were supported by public funds. These thoughts of Hitler's were not made public, but those physicians inclined toward Nazism, harboring similar notions, like Dr. Gerhard Wagner and Dr. Arthur Gütt, were advanced to key positions in the medical establishment after Hitler's rise to power. At one of the conferences of the Nazi Party in Nuremberg in the mid-thirties, Hitler and Wagner agreed that in the case of a war breaking out in Europe, this would provide the opportunity to rid Germany of all sorts of individuals considered inferior.

One more stage in preparing the ground for planned murder was in the appeal to SS officers who had fathered babies with defects to aid in their elimination. These officers had undergone Nazi indoctrination in SS academies, as had SS doctors. The SS press proclaimed in 1937 "no person had the right to act contrary to Nature and preserve the life of those who were not intended to survive." SS men were inculcated with the notion that those "of inferior value" had no justification to be an encumbrance on the living – even in the case of their very own children! In a well-known instance in 1938, an SS officer named Knauer[1] fathered a son with severe physical and mental disabilities. On the advice of the Nazi Prof. Werner Catel, director of the children's clinic at the University

1   Not everybody agrees about the identity of the baby involved. See Andreas Frewer and C. Eickhoff (Eds.). **"Euthanasie" und die aktuelle Sterbehilfe-Debatte.** Frankfurt and New York: Campus, 2000. pp. 120-143 [Ulf Schmidt].

of Leipzig, the parents turned to Hitler's chancellery with the request that their son be allowed to be put to death. Hitler asked his own personal physician, Dr. Karl Brandt, to examine the baby, who recommended that their wish be granted. From that date on, a strict watch was carried out in order to report the birth of babies with obvious disabilities. Midwives were offered special financial rewards when reporting the birth of a defective child to the authorities.

From here the path to compulsory euthanasia was short. The war drew near, and in the summer of 1939, during internal consultations within Hitler's chancellery, an added argument was raised: the necessity of clearing beds in institutions hospitalizing chronic patients – mainly the mentally ill – in order to make room for the benefit of those expected to be wounded in battle.

Activation of the Euthanasia order

On July 1939 Hitler empowered Leonardo Conti, the appointed Reich Health Leader, to organize the program of wide-scale planned medical murder. He provided him with two aides: his personal physician, Karl Brandt, together with Philipp Bouhler, an old-time Nazi lacking medical training who served as chief of Hitler's private chancellery. On August 10, the three assembled a team of twelve Nazi professors and physicians, chosen to serve in key positions in this deadly undertaking. Bouhler promised the group immunity from any possible legal prosecution, despite the fact that a law on this subject had not been officially legislated, the Nazis still fearing the reaction of world opinion, and even that of sections of the German public. The assembled physicians promised to cooperate and to keep silent. Participation in the killing project was not compulsory; a few physicians, such as Prof. Ewald of Göttingen, withdrew of their own accord, and did not suffer any repercussions as long as they kept the secret.

The only written basis for the euthanasia program was a five-line letter by Hitler, dated the day war broke out – 1 September 1939. It is now known that the date was a forgery; the letter was, in fact, written about two months afterwards. Presumably, the false date was designed to underscore the urgent nature of the action because of wartime.

Hitler's letter commissioned Bouhler and Brandt to designate physicians with the authority to euthanize patients: "so that a mercy death may be granted to patients who, in accordance with human judgment, are incurably ill according to the most critical evaluation of the state of their disease." This sanctimonious cover-up for the planned murder of tens of thousands was designed to mislead and mask the real nature of the operation. In addition, Hitler's letter was regarded as top secret: it was kept in a safe and taken out only for the sake of persuading physicians who showed qualms and demanded an official sanction for their actions. Later, in 1940 and 1941, proposals for a German state law were drafted, but were never adopted, the final legislation being postponed until an unspecified future date "after the victory."

The sterilization of chronic patients ceased during the war, the program became superfluous with the new policy of exterminating unwanted people. Nevertheless, there were cases where previously sterilized persons were put to death.

Immediately following the invasion of Poland, the first executions of the mentally ill took place, mostly of hospitalized Poles, but some of the patients were even of German origin (*Volksdeutsche*) who lived among the Poles. These patients, unlike the Poles, were given tranquilizing drugs before being killed, and were led to the site of execution one at a time, accompanied by SS soldiers in civilian clothes who talked with them to put them at ease. They were then dispatched by being shot from behind. These procedures of eliminating victims slowed down the process of murder and annoyed the directors of the operation in Berlin. Accordingly, the SS technical unit was charged with finding more efficient means of eradication. After various trials, carbon monoxide (CO) gas was selected as the agent of death, with the killing sites being deceptively disguised as bathrooms. The basements of six institutions for inmates throughout the Third Reich were outfitted for this purpose. The largest "death factory" was in Hartheim Castle, in the Oberdonau district of annexed Austria, near the birthplace of Hitler and Eichmann. In the course of one year, tens of thousands were put to death in this and other institutions[2] – nearly all of them Germans of **Aryan** descent.

---

2   Located in Bernburg near Dessau, Brandenburg near Berlin, Grafeneck in Württemberg, Hadamar in Hessen and Sonnenstein in Bavaria.

The administrative center for this deadly operation, in a spacious villa expropriated from its Jewish owners, was code-named T4, an abbreviation for its address in Berlin, Tiergartenstraße 4. Both the bureaucratic process and the liquidation procedure were uniform to all institutions. In the first stage of operations, tens of thousands of personal forms were sent to all institutions hospitalizing chronically ill patients. The institution directors were required to provide an assessment for each of their patients and the chances of their recovery. Some directors understood what was in the offing and did all they could to save their patients. It was possible to preserve some of them by claiming that they were of some use, as gardeners or librarians for instance.

The completed forms were returned to Berlin, to pass the classification of doctors who were in on the secret of Action T4. They quickly sealed the fate of the inmates after a perfunctory glance at the forms. The red pencil-mark "+" on the form sent the patient to his death. The procedure was speedy for a particular reason as well: the experts received the sum of only ten Pfennigs (about thirty cents in today's value) for each form turned over for their assessment. Thus in Nazi Germany, the total value of ten entire human lives, if they were considered of inferior value, amounted only to one single Mark! There were times when the doctors enlisted the help of their wives and mistresses in order to increase their income. In rare cases, the final judgment was referred to higher levels, mostly professors of psychiatry.

A special entry on the form specified the racial origin of the patients. In the case of Jews, even the pretence of medical consideration was mostly not kept, and they were condemned forthwith to death. However, the number of Jewish victims of Action T4 was not great. Most of them had been already been removed from the general health system and, in accordance with the Nuremberg Laws, were concentrated in Jewish institutions – which at this stage were, ironically, not included in the T4 program.

A special transportation company was designated to transfer the patients from the institutions to the liquidation centers. Buses of the German postal service were employed, with curtained windows to disguise their use. News of the planned end of the ride reached many of the patients, however, some of whom adamantly refused to go on the promised "excursion," and they had to be tranquilized or drugged with sleeping potions.

Upon reaching their destination, the patients were registered, photographed, and underwent a cursory medical examination. Only a few fortunate ones were saved from their dire fate. The rest were undressed and told that they had to undergo cleansing showers. They were led into a room in which plumbing installations gave it the semblance of a bathroom. When 70 to 80 patients were crowded into the room, a steel door was shut on them, and the doctor responsible for the process opened, with his own hands, the valves of the gas containers. After about fifteen minutes of great suffering, everyone was dead from asphyxiation. The doors were then opened and the corpses dragged out to the nearby crematorium. After the bodies had been cremated, the ashes were deposited in urns and given to the families upon payment.

The process of euthanasia was almost identical to the process of the killing of Jews in the extermination camps, which was put into effect at a later stage. In actuality, the T4 action served as a small-scale model for the mass genocide later on.

Thousands of disabled children (according to a rough estimate, about 5,000) were "mercy" killed under the brutal program, although the process in their case was more complex. The children were brought to university clinics, generally with the forced consent of their parents, and were examined by experts. Only after an authoritative decision that they had no chance for recovery were they put to death inside the clinics. The decision was made in accordance with the medical knowledge available at the time, with no consideration for the possibility that some could be successfully treated in the future. These children were not gassed to death, but were killed by overdoses of tranquillizers. The cause of death was falsified; their parents or guardians were informed that they had died of some disease.

The struggle over public opinion and the resistance to medical killing

As with the Holocaust, great efforts were made to camouflage the actions of T4 by the use of subterfuge and lies. After the victims had been killed, fictitious notifications were sent to their relatives, giving a false cause of death. From time to time, some embarrassing slips occurred: such as the report of a certain patient having died of appendicitis – when in fact, his appendix had been extracted years before. In another case, a woman received two notices in the same week of the death of her two retarded sisters, who had been perfectly healthy only a few days before. When she insisted that such a coincidence was unlikely, she was told the truth on the condition that she, being a faithful Nazi, would keep silent about it. However, others did not keep quiet. The "mercy killings" provoked considerable resistance. Soldiers returning from the front on leave were astonished to find that their retarded siblings had met an untimely death. Even in Nazi Germany, such an extensive operation could not be hushed up forever. Many of the victims had influential relatives. The many sudden death notices in newspapers gave rise to a spate of speculations. This was evidenced to the authorities by reports of public opinion among the German civilians, made by the Nazi security service (the SD) on a regular basis.

Among the Christian clergymen, a powerful opposition rose – a stark contrast to their later silence during the Holocaust. They opposed the T4 program both for religious reasons and because many of the fated victims, including children, were inmates of Church institutions. For example, there was an esteemed retarded children's village called Bethel, under the auspices of the Protestant mission who gave refuge to thousands of children and young people. The Institute's managing director, Pastor Friedrich von Bodelschwingh, refused to yield them to the T4 men. Bishop Clemens von Galen openly denounced the program in his Sunday sermons, and copies of the text of his Münster sermons were dropped by the Royal Air Force all over Germany.

Resistance from the Church finally forced Hitler in August 1941 to announce the termination of Action T4. By this point, 70,000 victims had already been killed. According to recovered documents, this was about the number the Nazis had originally intended to liquidate. One macabre document even calculated the financial benefit – to the last Pfennig – gained by the saving of food from the victims.

Most gassing installations in the death centers ceased operations as a result of Hitler's announcement – but the exterminations did not cease, they simply became subtler. The doomed patients, including many children, were starved to death or killed by lethal injections in the guise of beneficial medication. According to some sources, an additional 100,000 disabled persons, mostly mentally ill, were killed by these means by the end of the war. Others speak of an even larger number, up to 180,000 persons, bringing the human death toll of the so-called "Euthanasia" action to a quarter of a million people.

The Nazi propaganda machine made great efforts to try to legitimize the criminal acts of the medical personnel, either under the officially sanctioned Action T4 or the "wild" euthanasia following its cessation. Full-length films were produced during the war years designed to justify euthanasia. The most famous of them, **I Accuse** (*Ich klage an*), first screened in 1941, was an adaptation of a book written by a physician who participated in the children euthanasia program. The film, starring famous actors, was the story of a doctor demanding to put an end to the agony of his wife, formerly a talented pianist, afflicted with incurable, advancing multiple sclerosis. In it, she pleads desperately to be relieved of her suffering. The story in the film presents a typical case of a request for "mercy killing" in its humanitarian sense – but had no real connection with the compulsory medical murder of the helpless and unwilling victims of real or imagined hereditary diseases.

An additional shocking aspect of the euthanasia program was the claim that both living and dead victims served to benefit Science. Scholars of genetics and racial studies who, knowingly or not, collaborated, with the Nazis and their goals, wished to find, even in retrospect, a rationalization for their acts by dissecting some of the corpses for scientific research. For example, the staff of the Kaiser Wilhelm Institute for Brain-research in Berlin, which kept close ties with the extermination centre in nearby Brandenburg, took care to transfer about 500 brains of retarded victims to the Institute collection. Since the brains had to be extracted from the skulls immediately after death, a member of the Institute staff, Julius Hallervorden, stayed at Brandenburg to ensure the freshness of the anatomical research specimens. When asked to justify his involvement, he replied: "everyone here is destined to be killed anyway – and so at least they would also serve to the benefit of Science."

The shift from medical murder to genocide

It is likely that the official termination of the Action T4 in the summer of 1941 was occasioned also by the beginning of preparations for the "Final Solution" to the Jewish problem.

As already mentioned, the concentration of Jewish mental patients in Jewish institutes, according to the Nuremberg Laws, such as the large hospital in Sayn near Koblenz, spared their lives for a year or two. Sick Jews, who had been incarcerated in concentration camps, before these became extermination camps, were rounded up in the autumn of 1941 in a special operation code-named "14f13" and sent to their death by gas in the aforementioned Hartheim Castle.

With the invasion of the Soviet Union in the spring of 1941, a primitive method of mass murder was practiced at first; victims were shot in the back of the head and their bodies thrown into pits. Such a method was fraught with difficulties, however. Even hardened members of the special task forces (*Einsatzgruppen*) sometime balked at the task of massacring women and children.

At the end of October 1941, the directors of Action T4, whose operation had been temporarily suspended by Hitler's order, offered their services to the planners of the "Final Solution." In January 1942, almost at the same time as the Wannsee Conference, which approved the final plan to exterminate all European Jews, experienced operators of T4 were sent to the East. The chemist Helmut Kallmeyer met in Lublin with the high-ranking SS man Odilo Globocnik, and taught him the use of gas for exterminating people. Teams of T4 operators took part in the construction and operation of the first extermination camps in Chelmno, Belzec, Sobibór, and Treblinka. Dr. Imfried Eberl was appointed the first commander of the Treblinka death camp, after having gained experience in managing the T4 death institutions in Brandenburg and Bernburg. Other T4 doctors, wearing white smocks, oversaw the gassing of shipments of Jewish mental patients transferred to Chelmno from Germany, and continued afterwards to serve in the extermination of ordinary Jews.

The active participation of the T4 operators in the Holocaust completed the process of turning Nazi physicians into outright murderers. Even the most tenuous moral excuse – that of the need to liberate chronic patients from their suffering – was now removed. The scientists who had served in the program of eliminating Germans "of inferior value" were now conscripted to the continuation of Hitler's biological vision – the purging of the whole of Europe of the "racially inferior" Jews.

Had the Germans emerged victorious from the War, there can be little doubt that after the mission of exterminating all Jews had been completed, the Nazi leaders would have then returned to the task of racially purifying the German people themselves. Among the evidence for this is an official document of the German Ministry of the Interior, dated July 1940, in which all German nationals (non-Jewish!) have been divided hierarchically into four categories in accordance with their racial value. Most of those categorized in the lowest rank – a few millions – were considered unwanted. The Nazi biological vision would then have struck again, like a boomerang, against the German people themselves.

Further reading

Goetz Aly et al. **Cleansing the Fatherland; Nazi Medicine and Racial Hygiene.** Baltimore: John Hopkins University Press, 1994.

Henry Friedlander. **The Origins of Nazi Genocide; From Euthanasia to the Final Solution.** Chapel Hill and London: University of North Carolina Press, 1995.

Ernst Klee. **"Euthanasie" im NS-Staat; Die "Vernichtung lebensunwerten Lebens."** Frankfurt am Main: S. Fischer, 1983.

Hans-Walter Schmuhl. **Rassenhygiene, Nationalsozialismus, Euthanasie.** Göttingen: Vandenhoeck & Ruprecht, 1987, esp. pp. 178-260.

Chapter 5

The Berlin Jewish Hospital

The story of the Berlin Jewish Hospital and the plight of Dr. Walter Lustig, its director during the Nazi period, reflect and dramatize the unbearably cruel dilemmas confronting Jewish medical institutions of the time.

The beginning of the Jewish Hospital in Berlin dates to the middle of the eighteenth century, to the times of Moses Mendelssohn, the philosopher. In 1914 its complex of seven new buildings in the Wedding District of north Berlin were inaugurated, and it was in continuous use throughout the Holocaust.[1] The very dispersion of the hospital over separate buildings, as opposed to the one large building typical of many modern hospitals, was to be of importance later on.

This 200-bed hospital was built to the highest standards, and was provided with the finest equipment available at the time. Designed to serve Berlin's Jewish community, its regulations specified that it could treat patients of other religious denominations. Indeed, at the height of its activity, before the Nazi era, nearly half of its patients – either hospitalized or availing themselves of outpatient clinical services – were non-Jews. Because of its full patient capacity and the many private services provided, the hospital remained financially self-sufficient.

Several eminent physicians on its staff added to its renown: men like the kidney specialist Prof. James Israel, a highly-esteemed surgeon of impressive appearance, tall and bearded; and Prof. Hermann Strauss, who had managed the department of internal medicine for many years, and was eventually appointed director general of the hospital itself.

---

1 It is still in use today, under its old name, in the same quarter of Berlin.

The hospital at the beginning of the Nazi period

With Hitler's accession to power in 1933, the fate of the hospital changed drastically. Many non-Jewish patients were deterred from availing themselves of its services by anti-Semitic propaganda. After the Nuremberg Laws of 1935, the complete separation between Jews and non-Jews became state law. As a result, the number of hospital patients dwindled rapidly. The Jewish community was forced into massive financial support of the hospital. At the same time many of the Jewish patients themselves became destitute, as a result of the expropriation of Jewish property through the policy of Aryanization.

Many of the proficient staff of the hospital, in particular some of the younger physicians, foresaw the bleak Nazi future and left the hospital, some of them emigrating from Germany altogether. However, the vacancies were quickly filled by other physicians, who had been dismissed from other good hospitals in Germany.

Among those affected by the laws against Jews was the physician, Dr. Walter Lustig.[2] Born in a small town in Upper Silesia in 1891, Lustig studied medicine in Breslau. After his military service in World War I, he settled in Berlin in the twenties, marrying a non-Jewish physician, Annemarie Preuss. Lustig himself belonged to the broad stratum of assimilated Jews who saw themselves as Germans first and foremost, and whose connection with Jewish life was minimal. Politically, his tendency was towards the Right. In Berlin, his occupation was also not typical for a Jew: after having specialized in forensic medicine, he joined the police. Resourceful and diligent, he rose quickly to the head of the medical department of the Berlin police. This brought him into contact with Berlin persons of authority, and he became familiar with the ways of Prussian officialdom. The acquaintance and personal ties he developed during this period became useful during the Nazi era.

At the beginning of the Nazi reign, Lustig was dismissed from his position with the police, together with many other Jews in public service. Possibly due to his wife's unwillingness, he did not leave Germany, and

---

2   Daniel S. Nadav und Manfred Stürzbecher, "Walter Lustig" in: Dagmar Hartung von Doetinchem/Rolf Winau (eds.), **Zerstörte Fortschritte; Das Jüdische Krankenhaus in Berlin.** Berlin:Edition Hentrich, 1989.

earned his living in private work and in teaching at a nurses' training school.

In July 1938, all Jewish physicians in Germany, including Lustig, were struck with a great calamity: their licenses to practice medicine were revoked, and they could no longer work in their profession. Only a small group of Jewish physicians were allowed to continue medical practice: those who treated Jewish patients. The Jews remaining in Germany were still in need of medical services and, according to the race laws, Aryan doctors were not supposed to treat them. A few hundred Jewish physicians were enabled to take care of the Jewish population – but even then they were stripped of the respectable title of physician (*Arzt*), being known simply as *"Krankenbehandler"* (sick-carer). Even with this humiliation, such positions were much sought after.

Lustig, who had not been hitherto associated with the Jewish community, became now active in its affairs. His reasons were practical: seeking a new field of activity. He began to publish articles on medical subjects in the community periodical. Soon after, he became involved in the management of the community's health concerns. The man previously holding this position, Dr. Erich Seligmann, immigrated to the United States, and Lustig was appointed as his substitute after the *Kristallnacht* pogrom in November 1938. He was officially appointed "sick-carer," aided probably by his ties with the authorities and by his marriage to a non-Jewish wife. At that time, some of the senior physicians still remaining in the Berlin Jewish Hospital (like Chief of Surgery Dr. Siegfried Ostrowski) left their position, and Lustig attempted to find properly qualified substitutes for them.

The hospital at the time of transports to the East

In September 1939 the war broke out. Most of Europe was overrun by the invading Nazi forces, and the program of exterminating the Jews (the "Final Solution") was beginning to be put into effect. In October 1941, German Jews were beginning to be transported East, to concentration camps in Poland and (the lucky ones) to Theresienstadt. Dr. Lustig received an unusual appointment: he was put at the head of a committee of three physicians, operating under Gestapo auspices, with the task of reviewing the medical reasons for appeals of Jews against being transported.

At the time, the Jewish community of Berlin still numbered over seventy thousand, and many thousands of appeals piled up within a short time for the review of this committee. The committee convened inside the Jewish Hospital, where the necessary examinations also took place. Oddly, in accordance with the German principles of order, only the healthy Jews, at least in Germany, could be sent to extermination camps. Jews who were ill, or who were waiting to undergo operations, had first to be taken care of, in conformity with the stipulations of bureaucratic logic – and only upon their recovery to full health were considered fit enough to be sent to death.

Dr. Lustig and his colleagues carried out their serious duties faithfully. Their examinations were reliable and thorough, so that nobody was allowed to escape his fate of being sent East – unless he had genuinely cogent medical reasons. The Gestapo kept a strict watch over the actions of the committee and its members, checking their rulings from time to time.

Lustig responded well to the challenge of the Nazi authorities. Within eight or nine months, most of the work of the committee was done, and the major part of the Berlin Jewish population was uprooted – save for the lucky few who were considered unwell and were committed as patients to the Jewish Hospital. About ten thousand Jews, mostly young Jewish men and women, were left in Berlin to serve as forced labor in munitions plants.

In the summer of 1942, the time had come for Prof. Hermann Strauss, the director general of the hospital, to "retire." He had had the misfortune of not showing deference to an SS man, and not vacating his seat for him on the underground train. Owing to his advanced age and his respected position, Strauss was committed to the privileged ghetto in Theresienstadt. His place was filled, not surprisingly, by Lustig. This appointment in October 1942 was arranged by the Gestapo, the Jewish community having to approve it in retrospect, since the hospital was still, in theory, under its auspices. Bruno Blau, a cancer patient who was hospitalized for some years and was witness to what was happening at the hospital, remarked that the Nazis found in Lustig "a man after their own heart." His marriage to a non-Jew also garnered him favor in Nazi eyes. Even though this marriage had in the meantime proved unsuccessful, it should be noted that Annemarie Lustig understood that she couldn't initiate divorce proceedings against her husband. Had she done so, it would have shorn him of what little protection he may have enjoyed, with nothing to prevent him then from being sent to an extermination camp.

As head of the hospital, Lustig was highhanded in exercising his authority. This was born of the difficult circumstances. The staff had to show absolute obedience to every instruction from the Nazi authorities, including the wearing of the Jewish badge, the Yellow Star of David, even within the confines of the hospital. Fritz Wöhrn, a Gestapo man from Eichmann's department, was appointed by the Nazis to ensure that the orders were being carried out. He frequently used to pay sudden visits to the hospital and harass the workers. As one example, a nurse named Ellen Wagner was caught by him walking about without the Yellow Star, and was dispatched to Auschwitz the next day. Lustig did his best to cope with Wöhrn's evil nature. After the War, the minutes of Wöhrn's trial revealed the "cat and mouse" games with which Lustig often dodged him with admirable skill.

Lustig continually faced an overwhelming challenge – how to maintain the existence of the hospital in the face of both a Berlin Jewish community that was dwindling almost to nothing, and resistance from Eichmann and his staff, who sought to liquidate the institution, which in their opinion had lost its *raison d'être* with the elimination of the Berlin Jewry. Other directors of Jewish hospitals throughout the Third Reich faced similar dilemmas. The best known of them, whose conduct reminds one of Dr. Lustig, was Dr. Emil Tuchmann, the acting director of the Rothschild Hospital in Vienna, who had also been appointed by the Gestapo to manage an institution with which he had had no ties previously.

The threat to the continued existence of the hospital

At the end of February 1943, the action known as "*Fabrikaktion*" took place – the "cleansing" of Berlin munitions factories of their Jewish forced-labor. This was done on Goebbels' orders, intending to make Berlin free of Jews (*Judenrein*), in order to placate Hitler after the Stalingrad debacle that his forces had just suffered. On that day, Eichmann's men swept down on all the factories, rounding up their Jewish workers. Most of them were transported to Auschwitz a few days later.

A short time afterwards, on the dawn of the 10th of March, 1943, a long line of lorries assembled at the gates of the Jewish Hospital, with the orders to clear all the patients and the staff, and send them to the destined "Final Solution." On that day, Lustig made evident his ability and experience in dealing with authorities. Showing no overt signs of panic, Lustig demanded written instructions for the planned transportation. The embarrassed men, sent to carry out the mission, had brought with them no written orders – as Lustig had correctly guessed beforehand. In the meantime, Lustig got busy, contacting by telephone all his official acquaintances in order to rescind the decree. After a few hours, he succeeded; the lorries were forced to turn back empty, and the hospital was spared. The Gestapo accepted Lustig's argument that one Jewish hospital should be kept open in order to attend to the medical needs of the remainder of Berlin and Germany's Jews.

However, Lustig knew that the affair was not over. The Gestapo insisted on reducing the size of the hospital in accordance with its limited foreseen tasks. He was ordered to cut the staff within a day, by no less than fifty percent. Having to comply, he shut himself in over a restless night with his faithful secretary, Hilde Kahan, and his administrative aide, Erich Zwilski, in order to make the fateful decision about the names to be included on the list of those being sent East. The whole hospital was in an uproar. Nobody slept that night. Everybody understood all too well the meaning of what was taking place behind the locked doors, and the clatter of the typewriter dispelled any doubt. A list of about 300 names was finally signed, including also family members of several of the staff. The next morning, those on the list left for the assembly place for the East-bound transports. Some of them committed suicide.

Lustig tried to save the active professional nucleus of the hospital staff, particularly the experienced physicians and nurses, technicians and vital administration workers. But with all this, certain subjective considerations tainted his judgment, and gave rise to malicious rumors about him. He seemed to have given preference, for example, to those nurses whom he had befriended, during his separation from his wife, who was posted as a physician in distant Bavaria. There also were complaints that staff members who dared criticize his conduct found themselves on the evacuation list. Indeed, such occurrences had been common, and happened even later. The case of Dr. Carl Windmüller is documented, Lustig having added his name to one of the East-bound transports, in order to offer medical assistance during the journey to the patients evacuated from the hospital. Dr Windmüller had been critical of Lustig's conduct, and had also been involved an incident with the Gestapo inspector Wöhrn. It appears that Lustig was eager to get rid of him. Windmüller never came back. He is presumed to have been among those who perished in Auschwitz.

Some physicians who found they had lost favor with Lustig, or who had other reasons to fear for their lives, foresaw the coming blow, and to forestall it, simply went underground ("submerged," in the parlance of the times). Such was the case with Dr. Hermann Pineas,[3] the neurologist, who for six months managed the large psychiatric ward established in October 1942, for the hundred or so patients who had been transferred there from a Jewish institute in Sayn, near Koblenz. Pineas and his wife prepared their escape upon hearing of the impending clearing of all his patients. The Nazis saw no reason to keep Jewish mental patients alive, after having systematically sent to their deaths non-Jewish psychiatric patients in the framework of the T4 program. At the beginning of March 1943, Pineas and his wife were arrested for several hours by the Gestapo, ordered to vacate their lodgings and to report the next morning for deportation. That night they fled, and with the help of friends in Berlin and Vienna, found refuge in secret hiding places in Germany and Holland.

The hospital until the end of the war

The hospital survived the terrible crisis of March 1943, and continued to function until the end of the war. It took care of the hundreds of hospitalized Jewish patients, together with the remnants of the entire

---

3   Pineas's own story appears in Monika Richarz (ed.). **Jüdisches Leben in Deutschland; Selbstzeugnisse zur Sozialgeschichte 1918-1945.** Stuttgart: Deutsche Verlags-Anstalt, 1982. pp. 429-442.

German Jewry – several thousands, including Jews married to Aryan spouses (like Lustig himself) and their children who, though they were classed as *Mischlinge* (of mixed Aryan-Jewish parentage), were temporarily saved from extermination.

Towards the end of the war, the strict medical functions of the hospital became blurred with a broader function of survival, as shown convincingly by the Israeli historian, Rivka Elkin. The very necessity to continue treating patients in order to justify the existence of the hospital, coupled with the joint interest of staff and patients to prolong their stay as long as possible, thereby reducing the danger of their being sent East, encouraged instances of malingering and bogus treatment. Unwilling to get well, some patients declined to take medication, and some physicians aided in this subterfuge by prescribing unnecessary and time-consuming tests. These evasions often succeeded, despite the strict supervision of the authorities and of the hospital management.

A particularly severe moral dilemma facing the staff was the question of suicide. The number of suicide cases increased with the rising risk of transportation. The hospital entry registers recorded hundreds of attempted suicide cases. The large numbers provoked ethical questions among the staff. From a strictly professional viewpoint, a physician's duty was to preserve life. And yet, some thought it was preferable to let the patient die, thus saving him from the horrors of the extermination camps. Indeed, it was common for staff members not to overly exert themselves in order to save the life of a patient who had attempted suicide. Much caution had to be exercised in order to evade the watchful eyes of the authorities, who sought to reserve for themselves the privilege of determining the time of the death of their Jewish prey.

The medical function of the hospital became blurred for another crucial reason. In late 1943 Dr. Lustig was appointed as head of the representative organization for the remnants of the Jews of Germany, the "Reich Association of German Jews" (*Reichsvereinigung*). His good ties with the authorities undoubtedly helped him to obtain this additional but thankless position, a burden involving much toil and bother. Lustig carried out his duties almost by himself, in effect, a one-man Jews' Council (*Judenrat*), the mediating body between all remaining German Jews and the Nazis. He dealt with the welfare problems of the

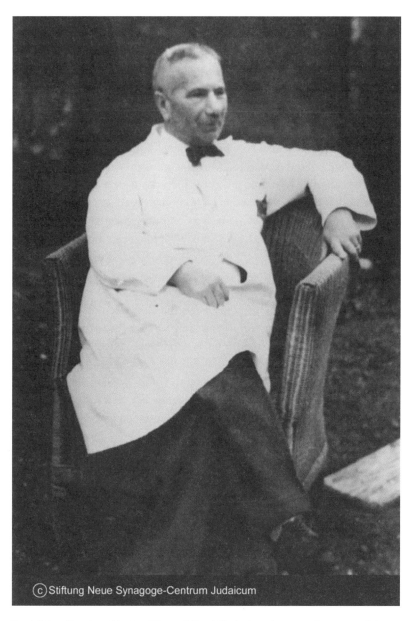

Dr. Walter Lustig with the "Star of David" during the war. Courtesy of Neue Synagoge Berlin – Centrum Judaicum.

last surviving Jews, with financial and legal questions, and with the management of the remaining Jewish assets.

Lustig's new role caused changes at the hospital. The offices of the Reich Association were housed in the hospital administrative wing, and its few workers were apportioned rooms in its offices. An even greater influence on the nature of the institution was the takeover of large sections for the benefit of German patients (mainly wounded soldiers), or for functions for which they had not been designed. The layout of the hospital facilitated this, divided as it was into seven separate buildings. The whole complex became a sort of microcosm, reflecting the demise of German Jewry. The nursing school had been expropriated long before to serve as a German auxiliary military hospital. This military hospital was later expanded to include what had been the obstetrics and gynecological building. Other buildings were taken over for completely non-medical uses: the former outpatient clinics were modified to serve the remnants of an evacuated Jewish old people's home. In another wing of the hospital, a workshop for the manufacture of children's clothing was established, employing some of the forced-labor workers who avoided, albeit only for a time, the transports East. In March 1944, the hospital's pathological institute, no longer in use for post-mortem operations, was turned into a "collection camp" (*Sammellager*) where Jews, such as those whose Aryan spouses had died, awaited a decision as to their fate under the watchful eyes of Gestapo guards.

The whole hospital, with its various remaining departments, was closely watched by the Gestapo, turning it into what Bruno Blau and others termed "the Berlin Ghetto." This ghetto suffered the continuous threat of raids by Wöhrn and other Gestapo men, who would drag people, the well and the ill, to their end.

However, there were also some positive aspects to this ghetto. In one of the former medical wards, dozens of children were sheltered, whose mothers claimed that they were the offspring of illicit affairs they had conducted with Aryan lovers, and therefore should be considered of mixed blood. It is in Dr. Lustig's favor – and even his detractors admit this – that he did his utmost to help these children, going so far as to enlist dubious witnesses in their defense in trials held to determine their paternity. In many cases, the protracted trials extended long enough to see some 90 of the children survive the war.

Dr. Lustig's end

Dr. Lustig himself, however, did not survive. During the lengthy battle over Berlin, most members of the hospital staff sheltered in the basement, and were saved from the bombardments and the shelling from Soviet tanks. The majority of the Jewish patients and prisoners survived the confusion of the final days of the Third Reich. The Berlin Jewish Hospital was the only place in all Berlin where Jews, some 800 in all, survived, with the acquiescence of the Nazi authorities. With the entry of the Russians into the hospital complex, they were greeted with unimaginable joy. Jews, at long last, were able to tear the hated Yellow Star from their clothes. Dr. Lustig offered to serve in a senior capacity in the health system the Russians were planning to set up, and suggested even to turn the "Reich Association," at the head of which he stood, into the infrastructure for the reorganized Berlin Jewish community. Then, however, his luck turned against him. After a few weeks, two Auschwitz survivors returned to Berlin and pointed Lustig out as the man who had sent them there after their recovery in the hospital. Lustig was arrested by the Russians, and without lengthy legal niceties, was put to death as a Nazi collaborator.

Thus ended the meteoric career of a Jewish physician, who, finding himself caught up in the flow of history and despite his best efforts, could not control its outcome.

The newly re-established Berlin Jewish community after the war was not proud of Lustig and his controversial actions. Even his photograph was not available for many years, until a distant relative of his was persuaded to donate a picture of him, wearing the Yellow Star, to an exhibition held in Berlin some years ago.

Some writers, such as Daniel Silver,[4] have tried to defend Dr. Lustig, but they rely mainly upon second-hand testimonies. It is impossible to get a clear and objective picture of the real man, his inner thoughts and his deeds during the war years. Lustig left no diary or other writings, which could enable us to penetrate the inner recesses of his soul. It is doubtful whether the ethical quandaries raised by his behavior, such as his surrendering of healthy people to their deaths, are answerable

---

4   **Refuge in Hell.** Boston: Houghton Mifflin, 2003 [German edition: 2006].

by those who have not been witnesses to the horrors of the Holocaust. These questions are part of the whole range of issues linked mainly to evaluation of the various *Judenrat* bodies during the Holocaust. On this matter, we should recall the ancient Jewish injunction against passing judgment on anyone – unless we have stood in his place.

Further reading

From Hekdesh to Hightec – The 250 year History of the Jewish Hospital Berlin. Berlin:Verlag für Berlin-Brandenburg, 2007 [a German version appeared at the same time].

Rivka Elkin. Das jüdische Krankenhaus in Berlin, 1938-1945. Berlin: Edition Hentrich, 1993.

Chapter 6

Theresienstadt

The Theresienstadt concentration camp, known in Czech as Terezin, was located inside a former fortress, built north of Prague by the Emperor Joseph II of Austria at the end of the eighteenth century and named after his mother, Maria Theresia. The fortress included extensive barracks for soldiers and small houses for officers and their staff, all surrounded by a wall. But its military use had been limited. At the beginning of the twentieth century, particularly in World War I, it had served to confine prisoners of war.

During World War II, the Theresienstadt fortress was converted by the Germans into a concentration camp for Jewish prisoners, to be considered a "model camp," having as its occupants some prominent persons such as Prof. Hermann Strauss, mentioned in the last chapter. However, all of this was organized so as to fool the world, and the Jews in particular, about the Holocaust in planning. Indeed, Theresienstadt contained no gas chambers, nor were there conditions of extreme hunger, as in other camps. The medical services there were of a relatively high level. But for all that, the Theresienstadt camp represented, in effect, an enormous deception – a presentation for the Red Cross and the rest of the world as the semblance of a "showpiece ghetto."

The reality behind the hoax, was that the Theresienstadt camp served basically as mere temporary quarters for Jews on their way to extermination. According to reliable statistics known today, which had been carefully hidden during the War years, some 144,000 Jews passed through the camp, but only 30,000 to 35,000 were allowed to remain there permanently. These were, however, mostly elderly people in their sixties and seventies, the mortality rate of whom was understandably high, exacerbated by the deplorable conditions and the impaired nourishment. Some of those who died in the camp, numbering 34,000, were replaced with other elderly prisoners. However, for most of the young and able prisoners, nearly 90,000, Theresienstadt was only a temporary stay, a transit station before they were sent out from there to extermination camps in the East, mainly to Auschwitz.

The beginning of Theresienstadt as a Jewish ghetto

After the German occupation of Czechoslovakia in 1939, the government of the Protectorate of Bohemia was somewhat more tolerant than that of occupied Poland later on. Members of the Prague Jewry (led by Jakob Edelstein) managed to convince the Nazi authorities, that incarcerating Protectorate Jews in Theresienstadt might serve as a better alternative to their transportation out of the country. In the autumn of 1941, young Jews, mostly volunteers, were sent to Theresienstadt from Prague and other communities, to prepare the camp to receive the prisoners intended for transportation. The aim was to make Theresienstadt a productive camp, where the inmates would work, thus convincing the Germans of their economic usefulness, and hence be allowed to survive. The enthusiastic young volunteers refurbished the rundown houses and barracks with their own hands, paved roads and fixed lighting.

At the end of November 1941, the first deportees arrived in the camp from Prague, and until spring 1942, the camp received some 30,000 Jews from all over the Protectorate and some elderly and prominent individuals from Germany. But at the same time, transports East were sent out from the camp. In January 1942, 2,000 Jews were relocated to Riga Ghetto – one of the worst. Almost all of them perished shortly after from starvation and cold. Thus began, in effect, a "revolving door" policy, an in-and-out movement of admitting Jews into the camp, on the one hand, and sending others from the camp to their extermination, on the other. The dream of those idealistic Jews who had regarded Theresienstadt as a place of refuge vanished from the start. The camp continued functioning until the end of the War – but in the ways the Nazis had always intended: ostensibly as a "model ghetto," having a Jewish self-administration, which enjoyed relatively extensive autonomy and was even allowed to mint currency for internal use and issue postage stamps. But in actuality, the camp served as a convenient assembling station for transports to extermination camps. And so, for example, 18,000 people were brought into Theresienstadt in September 1942 – while, at the very same time, 13,000 Jews were sent out from there to the East. In the autumn of 1942, this policy had reached horrific proportions, yet still remained undetected by the world outside.

The peak population of Theresienstadt came to some 58,500 (it had originally been intended for a full capacity of 11,000 soldiers in wartime). The overcrowding was extreme. This may explain, at least partially, the frighteningly high mortality rate – 3,941 people in September 1942 alone. According to available statistics, the area per prisoner at that time was only 2.2 square metres – comparable to the inhuman conditions of the Warsaw Ghetto. During 1943 the situation improved considerably, achieved at the grim expense of clearing some 20,000 inmates by having them sent to Auschwitz and other extermination camps. The immense overcrowding was most evident in the barracks, housing in one large hall several hundred men or women. Only later were the inner spaces there partitioned into rooms. Conditions in the separate and smaller houses were generally better. Some of these housed prisoners considered prominent or important: members of the intellectual and artistic elite of central and western Europe, or elderly Jewish veterans of the German army who had been awarded decorations in World War I.

Some of these privileged prisoners were even allowed to engage in artistic and intellectual pursuits. The cultural activities within the camp served as part of the subterfuge, disguising the real nature of "the town the Führer granted the Jews" – one of its frequent descriptions in the Nazi narrative. Theresienstadt was indeed noted for its cultural activities: plays, concerts, lectures, and the work of graphic artists and painters. Some artistically gifted physicians, such as Karel Fleischmann, managed to draw and document scenes from ghetto life, as well as to portray personalities, including their colleagues.[1]

Health and medicine in Theresienstadt

When the Germans set up the infrastructure of Theresienstadt, the vital importance of relatively good medical services was accepted

---

1 A collection of these works of art was published by the Israeli scholar, Dr. Tomi Spenser.

as self-evident. Part of this was also a certain obligation, which the legal-minded Germans did not take lightly: some elderly prisoners from Germany expelled to Theresienstadt were compelled to sign beforehand a document, whereby they agreed to give up all rights to their property – often amounting to large sums – for the benefit of the Nazis. In return, the authorities contracted to take care of their needs to their last days – including also complete medical care. This legally binding contract made it incumbent upon the Theresienstadt authorities to maintain, even in a partial way, the Nazi side of the agreement. Another factor was the availability of an enormous supply of Jewish physicians. No fewer than 720 physicians were imprisoned in Theresienstadt, amounting to one physician for some fifty persons – to this day a world record of doctors per capita! Even though some of the physicians had reached old age and left the practice of their profession, there remained a large enough reserve of able physicians to maintain an extensive medical service. Of the ghetto inmates, nearly one tenth was involved, in one way or another, in health services. This work had an important advantage: it granted all those employed in such services, the old and the young alike, immunity from being sent East. Only towards the end of the war, in the autumn of 1944, was this rule broken, and even physicians, including senior personnel, were sent to Auschwitz.

The patients in Theresienstadt were also treated in a way differing vastly from those in other concentration camps. Almost everybody who fell ill in Theresienstadt was free from the constant anxiety of such Jews in other camps, who knew that they were in immediate danger of being sent to the gas chambers in the next selection. The physicians in Theresienstadt were committed to curing their patients – and not to hastening their death, as Nazi doctors were ordered to do time and again, even in the case of their own German brethren. Only two groups of patients were treated differently in Theresienstadt: the mentally ill and the tubercular. Several hundreds of such patients are known to have been gathered and sent to Auschwitz in several transports.

Most patients in Theresienstadt received some medical response to their complaints, from minor care such as headache pills to relatively complex surgery, undertaken routinely in the ghetto hospitals. Even orthopedic shoes were made in Theresienstadt, together with artificial limbs and eyeglasses manufactured in special workshops. Despite all this, the horrendous overcrowding, the meager diet, the poor hygienic conditions and even the scarcity of water took their toll, neglecting the preventive aspects of medicine, the basis of all reasonable health care. These and other factors aided the spread of disease, and demanded energetic actions to combat their inevitable result. They could be ignored neither by the camp authorities, nor by the Jewish self-governing council.

The heads of the health services at Theresienstadt

The highly reputed Jewish physician, Dr. Erich Munk, was the director of the ghetto Department of Health from its start. He was competent both as a clinician and as an administrator. There are contradictory assessments of him as a person. On the one hand, noted ghetto historian Hans Adler described him in uncomplimentary terms. Under different circumstances, in Adler's opinion, Munk undoubtedly could have been successful. In the ghetto, however, because of his overbearing personality and the sense of haughtiness in his dealings with most people who worked under him, he could not obtain the collaboration needed for dealing with the difficult conditions. On the other hand, the dermatologist, Dr. Karel Fleischmann, who served as his deputy and managed the Welfare Section of the Department of Health, described another aspect, one of warm compassion – for example, with regards to children – and even a sense of humor. It seems that Fleischmann was one of the few who managed to get along with him. But generally it is apparent that there could have been better cooperation among the staff members.

Dr. Munk behaved in a dictatorial manner, wielding his authority whether necessary or not. All this aside, however, he was a dedicated and hard-working man. In a letter in 1942, Dr. Fleischmann described Munk when new transports were arriving daily at the ghetto gates:

> Dr. Munk worked day and night. In July he slept really only a few hours. And even when retiring to his bed, he had to think about what would happen on the morrow… I often came early to the office and found him at his desk. On answering the question why he began his day so early, he replied that he had not gone at all to sleep…

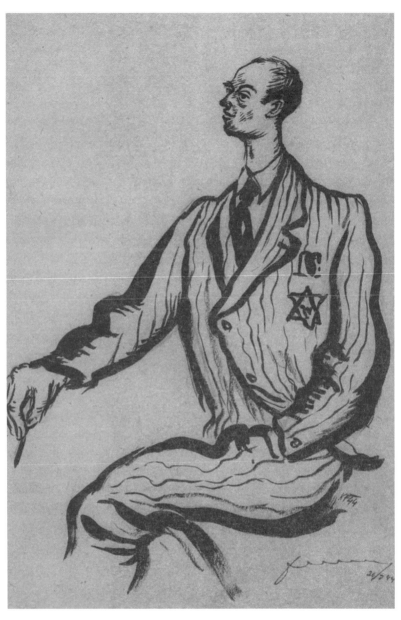

Dr. Erich Munk. (Drawn by Dr. Karel Fleischmann). Courtesy of Yad Vashem Art Museum.

Some of Munk's efforts were not well directed. His door was not open to those responsible for the many units within the health system; all relations with them were maintained through written orders only. Munk used to explain this as the necessity to document every action for the benefit of the German overseers, who relied on him and allowed him considerable freedom of action. However, it seems that after some time and for reasons unknown, Dr. Munk fell out of favor with the Germans and was sent to the extermination camp in the autumn of 1944. His devoted deputy, Dr. Fleischmann, met a similar fate. Both men perished in Auschwitz. Notwithstanding Munk's shortcomings, a fully functioning, extensive and decentralized medical system was developed in the ghetto, which adapted itself well to the special conditions of the patients. Most needy patients, not surprisingly, were elderly people. Hans Adler stated that through frequent medical attention, an aging prisoner would find a way to obtain some benefit: a glass of milk or one more slice of bread. It must be remembered that though there was no real starvation in Theresienstadt, nutrition was poor, averaging in 1942 only about 1,600 calories per day per person. Those who did not work – i.e., most old people – received even less. All prisoners lost weight and were also forced to reduce smoking to a minimum because of the extremely limited supply of cigarettes. Some physicians, like Dr. Reis, noted the positive consequences of this condition; but, on the other hand, the unbalanced diet, with its paucity of proteins and sugars, was often the cause of severe digestive disturbances and gastric complaints.

There were almost no means of transportation in the ghetto, and some patients were totally bedridden. This necessitated the operating of many dispersed clinics and small rooms for the sick (*Krankenstuben*) adjacent to the living quarters of most prisoners, especially in the large barracks. Several clinics and hospitalization units were active at the same time including some units for the isolation of patients suspected of carrying contagious diseases.

A situation report from September 1942 lists the existence of no fewer than 438 sick rooms in the ghetto, with a capacity of almost 5,000 beds. In addition, there were also fourteen isolation rooms with seventy beds. Thirty-six additional clinics treated patients before having them hospitalized for more extensive treatment. All these smaller units were well dispersed throughout the living quarters. The physicians and other medical staff were also ready to attend to anybody who could not reach

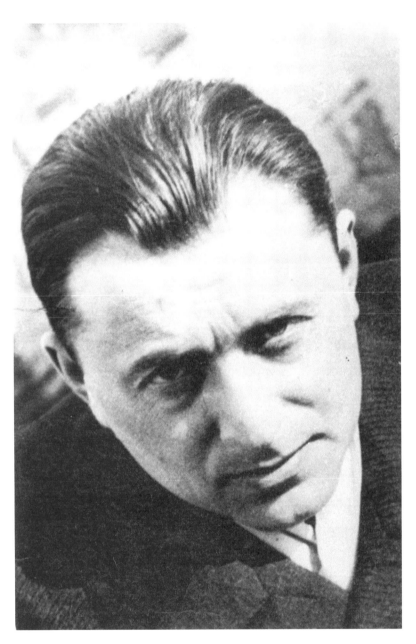

Dr. Karel Fleischmann. Courtesy of Yad Vashem Archives.

the sick-rooms on his own. These frequent house calls were only possible because of the large number of medical workers.

The Theresienstadt medical system incorporated several central institutes, including a general hospital equipped with a large surgical ward, a hospital for respiratory illnesses, an infectious diseases hospital, and even a small children's hospital. The ghetto also had an X-ray institute and well-equipped laboratories. Nonetheless, there were periods when the medical staff found it difficult to withstand the pressure of the many in need. Patients crowded the doors of clinics and sick rooms and were not always able to be treated well. In one instance, in February 1943, the number of all patients neared one third of all Theresienstadt prisoners. Even in this case, however, the mortality rate remained reasonable: 79 dead – two-tenths of a percent of the population – an astonishingly small figure, bearing witness to the success of the treatment in spite of the heavy work load.

The medical equipment and store of medications at Theresienstadt were usually acceptable in quality, though in the initial days of the ghetto, the medical staff were tried by many severe difficulties. We have on record a case of an urgent leg amputation performed in a bathroom with a carpenter's saw. Dr. Benno Krönert, the German physician appointed by the camp administration – who appears to have been relatively accommodating – acted energetically towards the acquisition of needed medical supplies. These were taken in part from Jewish hospitals in Germany, which the Nazis had shut down, confiscating their equipment. After a year or two, difficulties arose in obtaining certain medications, in particular sulfa drugs needed at the Front. Occasionally the Council of the Elders (as the *Judenrat* of Theresienstadt was called) was able to procure them at great cost, or even illegally, particularly if they were essential to the treatment of some prominent prisoners whom the Germans desired to keep alive.

Theresienstadt Ghetto served as a concentration camp for many young Jews prior to their expulsion to the East, including families with young children. This occasioned many instances of pregnancies amd births. A small children's hospital enabled mothers to give birth, and their children received care in a special clinic when in need. It is estimated that 230 babies were born in Theresienstadt, nearly all of whom perished, following the transport of many families to Auschwitz in the autumn of 1944. Only about twenty children born in Theresienstadt survived the War. One of these few (Michael Wiener) was to serve in the mid-1990s as the chief medical officer of the Israeli army.

Diseases in Theresienstadt

Among the common afflictions of the camp inmates were diseases of the alimentary tract, particularly colitis and enteritis. The latter was the most common cause of death: some 8,500 deaths during the operation of the camp. The spread of intestinal diseases was caused in part by poor diet and in part by the deteriorating mental state of inmates. Gastric ulcer was also of common occurrence at Theresienstadt. Other widespread diseases were pneumonia – that infamous common killer of old people – which caused over 6,000 deaths, and also heart diseases and infections. One phenomenon typical to Theresienstadt was the outbreak of children's diseases, such as measles or mumps, among the adult population. Experts explain this as a result of a widespread mental regression occurring among the aged. About twenty cases of infantile poliomyelitis among adults were diagnosed as well, occasioning a special study.

The bodies of the many dead in the ghetto were cremated. Some of them, chiefly of religious Jews, were buried in a cemetery outside the camp.

The assembly of numerous physicians in Theresienstadt, some of who were eminent specialists, together with the relative liberty for cultural activities allowed by camp authorities (albeit for their own reasons), facilitated the possibility of self-improvement and even of medical research. When Prof. Herman Strauss, the retired former head of the Berlin Jewish Hospital, arrived at Theresienstadt in the middle of 1942, he organized a system of refresher courses and studies for the medical personnel. A list survived, reflecting these activities during the short period of two weeks in the summer of 1943. In that period, twenty lectures were held, covering all medical fields, as well as symposia and discussions among the physicians. Organized rounds in hospitals were held to gain experience from medical cases of interest – a common practice in most modern medical institutes. Some of the lectures were open to the general public, and stressed particular aspects of preventive medicine, such as the combating of vermin and lice.

Some of the experts in Theresienstadt were noted chemists, such as Arthur Eichengrün, the co-inventor of aspirin. Although married to an Aryan, he was sent to the ghetto because he had omitted in some document the middle name "Israel," which all male Jews in Germany were forced to add to their names. He remained in Theresienstadt from the beginning of 1944, and in spite of his advanced age of 76, worked in a relatively well-stocked laboratory in the camp, producing several medications that were scarce owing to war conditions.

A collection of reports of scientific studies undertaken by Jewish physicians at Theresienstadt were gathered and deposited in Israel's Yad Vashem archives by Dr. Marc Dvorjetski, himself a survivor of Vilnius Ghetto and Estonian labor camps.[2] These reports of studies, though less extensive than those from the Warsaw Ghetto, are still of value. Notable examples include those on the widespread phenomenon of anemia in the Theresienstadt Ghetto, due to a diet deficient in iron and proteins. Other studies dealt with poliomyelitis and with meningitis, a disease that afflicted some 1,000 persons in the ghetto, particularly children, provoking great alarm.

Some of the studies were aided by the findings of post-mortem autopsies, which were frequently carried out in Theresienstadt. There are reports of around 150 such procedures, some of which were performed in order to assess the reasons for the failure of more complex operations in the central hospital. Such procedures were similar to those carried out in established institutes. The conclusion was that frequent failures were occasioned by the interruption of electricity in the camp. The absence of telephone communication and vehicles, to obtain outside help, also contributed to these failures.

Most of the surgical procedures, nevertheless, were successful. Some of the physicians survived the War and came to Israel. Dr. Richard Stein, the noted ophthalmic surgeon, saved the eyesight of hundreds of patients at Theresienstadt. Some of his patients were high-ranking Nazi officers, who threatened his life were the operations to fail. On coming to Israel in 1948, he was immediately made a member of the staff of a new military hospital in the Tel Aviv area, and quickly rose to become head of the ophthalmic section. Continuing his work, he is credited with saving the eyesight of many in Israel.

It would seem proper to end with one final quotation from the writings of the deputy director of the Theresienstadt Department of Health, Czech-born Dr. Karel Fleischmann, who perished in Auschwitz in 1944. His writings and drawings are preserved at Beit Terezin, in Kibbutz Givat Haim in Israel. Dr. Fleischmann's tone is understandably pessimistic. In

2   His life and work will be dealt with in Ch. 10.

spite of the impressive achievements of health workers at Theresienstadt, the circumstances were such that even the most dedicated struggle would not, or could not, emerge victorious in the final count. The vast majority of the prisoners died or were exterminated sooner or later, whether in Theresienstadt itself (only some 19,000 finally survived that camp[3]) or in the death camps. Dr. Fleischmann's anguished words still echo today:

> Tomorrow another hundred dead will be added. Tomorrow the pharmacy, called "The Central Store of Medications," will issue another large amount of preparations, meant presumably against cardiac pain. Tomorrow, God, another multitude of the "purified" will stand before Thy throne of glory. And I continue on... But I do not know what Theresienstadt is. It is a splendid terror. It is a struggle of white corpuscles against fever. It is an enormous field hospital, next to the front, disturbed by the din of battle taking place nearby. It is a modern, flexible and mobile organisation, capable of performing [but] without means of transportation, without telephone, without bicycles... and even the electric supply is conditional... Another day passed. What day? Even not one second... Whither, whither does Time gallop like a madman, for those candidates for death?

Further reading

H.G. Adler. **Die verheimlichte Wahrheit; Theresienstädter Dokumente.** Tübingen: J.C.B. Mohr, 1958.
Ruth Bondy. **"Elder of the Jews," Jakob Edelstein.** London: Grove, 1989.
Zandek Lederer. **Ghetto Theresienstadt.** London, 1953.

---

3   Including two groups of prisoners who were freed and sent to Switzerland and Sweden towards the end of the war; 3,000 others survived Auschwitz.

Chapter 7

Warsaw Ghetto

With the Nazi conquest of Poland in September 1939, the Germans took over a territory, home to some three million Jews, in a very short time. Of these, about a million lived in the eastern part of Poland, which had been occupied by the Russians for two years, in accordance with the partition agreement made before the War between Germany and the Soviet Union. During the two years of Russian occupation, some of the Jews – who were fortunate enough – were exiled to inner parts of Russia on the suspicion of being a Zionist, or were drafted into the Red Army. Most, however, once again found themselves under Nazi reign with the German invasion of the Soviet Union in the spring of 1941.

Ghettoization in Warsaw and the role of German physicians

When the Nazis conquered Poland, they were troubled with the question of what to do with the millions of Jews who had fallen into their hands. At this time, the decision to annihilate all the Jews had yet to be reached. Suggestions had been made to deport them to Madagascar or concentrate them within a limited zone on the Polish eastern border. The eventual plan, executed in only a few months, and, in the case of Warsaw, after one year of occupation – was ghettoization. In effect, this meant the imprisonment of Jews within a well-defined, fenced-in area in each of the cities or towns that had had a significant Jewish population before the War.

The governor of occupied Poland, Hans Frank, was the plan's chief instigator; and it was implemented by Reinhard Heydrich, commander of the Nazi Security Service (SD), who also served as the chairman of the Wannsee Conference (20 January, 1942). Nazi physicians played a central role in this undertaking. The involvement of Nazi doctors like Jost Walbaum and Josef Rupprecht has been revealed by the research of Christopher Browning,[1] among others. Immediately following the Nazi conquest of Poland, Walbaum and Rupprecht expressed the view that the Jews were the bearers of germs and diseases, and needed be isolated from the rest of the Polish population, the hygienic conditions of which they considered deplorable anyhow. This presumed Polish neglect of basic hygiene conformed with the general perception of Nazi physicians that Poles and the Slavs generally were of an inferior status to Aryan Germans. The Jews were placed in an even lower position in the hierarchy. In Nazi eyes, Jews thus acquired the reputation as disease carriers and epidemic spreaders, just as they had during the Black Plague in the Middle Ages. These views were even published in a presumably scientific volume prepared in occupied Poland during 1941.[2]

Needless to say, such accusations were utterly groundless. Even though much of the Jewish population lived in dire poverty, the hygiene among them was generally good; this was due to their kosher dietary laws and the religious requirement of purification. Jewish communities were concerned with fostering measures of hygiene, sanitation and preventive medicine. Organizations such as TOZ (*Towarzystwo Ochrony Zdrowia*), the Society for the Protection of Health of the Jews, established in 1922, were active in this sphere. Those organizations were aided financially by private individuals and organizations such as the JDC (Joint Distribution Committee of American Jews). TOZ undertook, for example, mass inoculations against tuberculosis and other diseases.

All throughout Poland, numerous Jewish hospitals and clinics were in operation, sometimes better equipped than the medical facilities available to the general population. In the traditional Jewish spirit of mutual responsibility, the Jewish communities offered medical care for the ill, often for free, with the aid of voluntary fraternal associations. As a result, the morbidity rate among the Jews was significantly lower than for the rest of the Polish population. Such a reality did not hinder the Nazi anti-Semitic propaganda, continually comparing the Jews – even by graphic means such as the German film "The Eternal Jew" – to vermin and rats.

---

1   "Genozid und Gedunheitswesen; Deutsche Ärzte und polnische Juden 1939-1941," in: **Der Wert der Menschen; Medizin in Deutschland 1918-1945.** Berlin: Hentrich, 1989. pp. 316-328.

2   J. Walbaum (ed.). **Kampf der Seuchen – Deutscher Ärzte-Einsatz im Osten.** Krakau: Buchverlag, 1941.

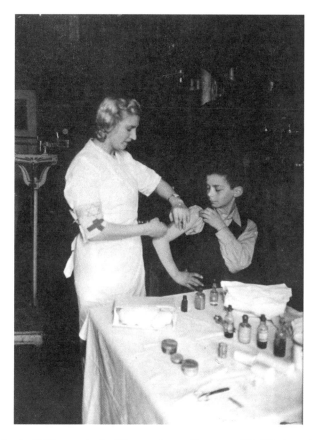

Inoculation by TOZ nurse in the Warsaw ghetto. Courtesy of Yad Vashem Archives.

Within the first year after the German occupation, the Jewish morbidity rate had indeed increased (though it had not yet reached epidemic proportions): the direct result of the occupation itself and the constant persecution. Even prior to the ghettoization of the Jews, their livelihoods were hampered, reducing their income, in turn influencing their nutrition – with negative effects on immunity and resistance to disease. Despite the obstacles, it appears the communities were still able to deal with the health problems they faced, and managed to take care of sanitation and preventive medicine. Jews who were forcibly exiled from their previous homes and sought shelter from Nazi persecution (for example, after having been expelled from the sizeable territories annexed to the German Reich), were generally well received, integrated into their new Jewish communities and provided with medical care.

These facts were not sufficient to convince Walbaum, who argued that the Jews are the chief natural carriers of spotted typhus and that their shifting from place to place facilitated the spread of this disease all over Poland. He and other Nazi physicians warned of a potential epidemic, which could debilitate the German forces and administrative personnel governing occupied Poland. They argued that Germans lacked the presumed natural immunity, which the Jews had acquired over generations of exposure to the illness endemic among them. They ignored the fact that there were no typhus epidemics among Jews at the time, thanks to the effectiveness of their preventive measures. The general demonization of the Jews by the Nazis hindered the Nazi doctors from an objective assessment of the facts.

When a sole German physician, Dr. Nauck, voiced a heterodox opinion – that the diet and living conditions of the Jews should be improved he was unquestioningly rejected. The idea of a humane attitude towards Jews contradicted the basic beliefs of most Nazi doctors. For them, the contrary was true: these physicians, who were the pioneers and standard bearers of the ghettoization, saw the solution as a logical continuation of the accepted medical strategy of combating epidemics through the isolation of disease-bearing individuals. The German physician responsible for public health, Kurt Schrempf, was empowered to determine if the Jewish schools could be opened, in view of their supposed sanitation problems. He decided to leave them closed.

Nazi leadership readily accepted the idea of ghettoization. The strategy was, in their eyes, helpful in the continued humiliation and harassment of the Jews. Heydrich and others, anticipating the Final Solution, ordered ghettos to be established in large cities, near central railroad connections. Concentrating Jews in such ghettos would ease their transfer to the sites of mass extermination when the time came.

Already by the end of 1939, suggestions to incarcerate Jews in a ghetto in Warsaw, the largest Jewish concentration in Europe, had been made. Disagreements among German authorities postponed putting the plan into effect until November 1940. Initially the Germans encircled most of the Jewish neighborhoods in Warsaw with a barbed-wire fence,

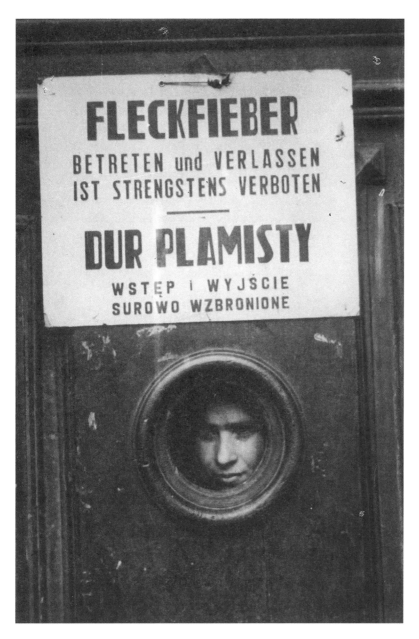

A warning in Warsaw ghetto: Spotted fever. Entry and exit strictly forbidden.
Courtesy of Yad Vashem Archives.

with signs stating: "Warning! Danger of Epidemics. Entry Forbidden!"
This was clearly the influence of Nazi physicians and the beginning
of a process, which can best be termed: "the medicalization of the
Holocaust."[3]

In November 1940, an area designated to be the ghetto was
enclosed by walls (some of them temporary), eighty thousand Poles
were cleared out and no less than 140,000 Jews were forced into
the area. In a matter of weeks they were all crowded in with several
tens of thousands of Jews who already lived there. Within the next
few months, a further 150,000 Jews were driven into the ghetto. At
its most crowded stage, in April 1941, the Warsaw ghetto numbered
450,000 people. The overcrowding was horrendous. One-third of the
population of the entire city of Warsaw (plus numerous refugees from
the outside) was crammed into the ghetto, which took up no more than
three-four percent of the built area of the city. People were crowded
seven to a room. The ghetto was in the poorest vicinity of Warsaw; the
problems exacerbated by the run-down environment, cramped streets
and deficient drainage.

Health and medicine in the Ghetto

The medical infrastructure within the ghetto was improvised. The large,
modern Jewish hospital of Warsaw in Czyste built before the war, had
been left outside the ghetto boundaries. With great difficulty, the *Judenrat*,
headed by the engineer Adam Czerniakow, managed to extricate from it
some supplies and equipment, and established in the ghetto subsidiary
branches of the abandoned hospital. These were located in poorly-built
houses, utterly unfit for their new function.

Despite the adverse conditions, the ghetto health department, headed
by Dr. Israel Milejkowski, tried its best to improve the situation. Every
effort was made to provide medical treatment for the needy by a vast
extension of the public health sector (the rich – and there were some in

3   "The medicalization of the Holocaust" defines the process of medical involvement
     in the annihilation process. Christopher Browning spoke already in similar terms at
     a conference in Berlin, November 1988. His written text appeared in **Der Wert der
     Menschen** (1989), as mentioned before. See also the details of his important later
     book at the end of this chapter.

the ghetto – were treated privately). A supervising board of physicians oversaw the activities and reported directly to the *Judenrat*, which spent one third of its budget on medical and sanitary needs. At the height of ghetto activities, there were two hundred physicians in public service, two hospitals operating in six different buildings, three outpatient clinics and eight neighborhood disinfection units. While the United States had not yet joined the war, the JDC continued contributing funds for health purposes, and preventive measures, such as inoculations and chest X-rays.

The *Judenrat* acted energetically to improve sanitation in houses and surroundings as well. Every house had an appointed committee with sweeping powers which the dwellers were required to obey. Inhabitants maintained a rotation of tasks such as cleaning the yards and the stairs, and collecting the refuse and its disposal. In houses and streets suspected of being infected with germs or open diseases, all dwellers were gathered in order to carry out collective disinfections. Their clothes were steamed in order to be rid of vermin; their bodies were washed with antiseptic soap and bathed in warm water. Even in mid-winter, these disinfecting actions were carried out, with steam cauldrons in the open – sometimes an invitation for respiratory diseases. The vacated dwellings were likewise disinfected. After forty-eight hours, the people were allowed to return. In spite of all the difficulties, these measures proved effective in combating epidemics, especially typhus (which is transmitted by rodents and vermin). Even members of the Jewish criminal underworld had a role: they donated their particular skills to the health efforts, managing to smuggle into the ghetto essential medicines, and even an ambulance.

In 1940, the Warsaw morbidity rates were only a little higher than the pre-war statistics. In 1941 and the first half of 1942, however, a continuous increase in the number of illnesses and deaths was recorded, in spite of all the preventive measures. In a terrible irony, the substandard dietary, hygienic and medical conditions in the ghetto fulfilled the Nazi physicians' predictions: diseases and epidemics began to spread through the Warsaw ghetto. The rising mortality rate was due mainly to starvation. By the end of 1941, close to 4,500 deaths per month were recorded – more than one percent of the ghetto population. At such a rate, the ghetto would have been liquidated within eight years, without the need for extermination camps – but for the Nazis, this was too long to wait.

The terrible scarcity of food was such that whoever relied only on official handouts had to make do with only one tenth of the amount of calories needed for survival. The *Judenrat* opened free public kitchens, which provided one meager meal a day for the needy – but this was far from sufficient to halt the humanitarian disaster. The body's weakened natural immunity was not capable of withstanding the onslaught of microbes and germs. Many died of disease: pneumonia, tuberculosis and abdominal diseases. Without wood many simply froze to death in the harsh winters. Photographs of dead children lying frozen in the streets of the ghetto still haunt us.

The German health authorities were not troubled at all by the mounting death rate in the ghetto. Only one German physician, the former Socialist, Wilhelm Hagen, proposed improving the ghetto food rations as a means of combating epidemics – but he was removed from his post before long. Many Germans were overjoyed to read the grim death statistics. On the other hand, however, the beginning spread of epidemics, such as spotted typhus – about two thousand cases in a few months – were a source of worry. The disease spilled from the ghetto walls, and all brutal, stringent German efforts to tighten the siege could not truly seal the ghetto off hermetically. Furthermore, German soldiers had to be present within the ghetto, and were thus exposed to health hazards. The Germans were forced to recognize the need for disinfection and a more active resistance to the spread of disease, which had begun to endanger also Poles and even German families beyond the ghetto walls.

The "faculty of medicine" within the Ghetto

In view of these circumstances, the Germans acceded to the *Judenrat* suggestion to establish within the ghetto two courses for sanitation. Thus an opportunity was gained to maintain a clandestine medical school in the ghetto, which operated undiscovered for a year and a half under Nazi eyes.

In the ghetto there were hundreds of idle Jewish medical students who had been compelled to abandon their studies in Polish universities following the German conquest. Dozens of Jewish lecturers in medicine lost their posts as well and were forced into the ghetto. A Polish professor of medicine in the University of Warsaw, anatomist Eduard Loth, maintained his ties with his young Jewish assistant incarcerated in the ghetto, Ludwig Stabholz, who was a scion of a famous family of physicians. His uncle, Henryk Stabholz, served as head of surgery in the branch of the Czyste hospital, transferred to the ghetto, and perished in March 1941 as a result of an infection contracted in the course of his work.

According to L. Stabholz,[4] Loth persuaded the *Judenrat* to take advantage of German permission to hold courses in sanitation, in order to maintain an active medical school within the ghetto. He also assembled a secret session of the Faculty of Medicine council at the University of Warsaw, which decided to recognize some of the courses of study held in the ghetto. At this meeting, the council granted the rank of professor to a few Jewish lecturers, including the thirty-one-year-old Stabholz, This would allow the university to formally accredit the marks they gave their students.

The existence of this unique institute, a ghetto medical school, is an impressive testimony to the resoluteness of its students and lecturers, who defied the Nazi attempts to extinguish Jewish intellect. The staff of this institute trained some five hundred students, one-tenth of whom survived the Holocaust to continue their studies. Many of the lecturers – some of whom were involved in research too – perished at the hands of the Nazis.

Dr. Milejkowski apportioned funds for the printing of instructional material, and the *Judenrat* allocated an abandoned secondary school building for the studies. The site was near the ghetto walls and the proximity of the German patrols necessitated strict measures of security and secrecy. Formulas for disinfection were always inscribed on the blackboards and the floor was strewn with disinfecting powders in an attempt to camouflage the true nature of the instruction.

Well-known lecturers, like Professor Ludwik Hirszfeld, the serologist,[5] and Julius Zweibaum, who taught zoology, headed the

---

4   L. Stabholz was interviewed by the author a few times in his Tel Aviv apartment before his death in 2007 at the age of 96.

5   Ludwik Hirszfeld made a name for himself in World War I, according to Charles Roland's study (p. 194), by defining "Salamonella hirszfeldi." Hirszfeld, who converted to Christianity, continued to visit the only church in the ghetto every Sunday, even while confined there. He escaped to the Aryan side in 1943 and survived the war.

Faculty. The curriculum consisted of two central courses, in accordance with the level of study reached by the students prior to their being expelled to the ghetto. First- and second-year students were taught basic disciplines such as biology, chemistry, anatomy and histology, in accordance with the curriculum of the University of Warsaw. Prof. Loth managed to smuggle into the ghetto professional literature and preparations essential to the academic study of the two latter subjects, taught by Dr. Stabholz. The second, more advanced course dealt with clinical subjects and specializations. Final-year students interned in the ghetto's makeshift hospitals. Their specialization was mostly in name only. Without even minimal conditions, equipment and medications, it was almost impossible to do real medical work.

Hunger research

Within the medical school, and with the aid of experts outside, a unique study was held in the Warsaw Ghetto on the medical results

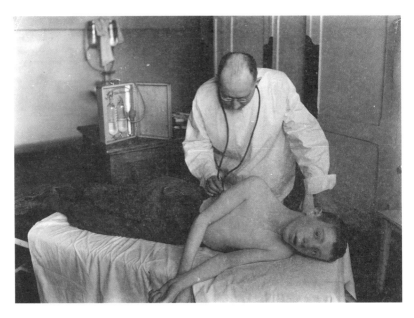

A physician (probably Dr. Zweibaum) examines a patient in the Warsaw ghetto. Courtesy of Yad Vashem Archives.

of malnutrition. This scientific research – evidence that the traditional Jewish reverence for scholarship could not be extinguished even under these adverse circumstances – has lasting value today.

Seven teams of physicians participated in the research, examining the results and implication of starvation. Each specialized in investigating the effects of hunger on one of the systems of the human organism. The researchers included people renowned in their field, such as the internist Julian Fliederbaum, and the cardiologist Emil Apfelbaum. Many others, like Dr. Symcha Lederman, who perished later in Treblinka, assisted to the best of their abilities. The study was conducted according to strict scientific methodology. Human subjects for the study were, of course, to be found in abundance. The participants occasionally received one or two slices of bread after their examinations, as a reward for their cooperation. To serve as a control group, the testers made use of members of the criminal underworld (who contrived means to stay well-fed even in the conditions of the ghetto).

The study investigated the effect of hunger on the development of children and adolescents, on the metabolism, on eyes and vision, on blood vessels and the heart, and on the digestive system. The faculty of medicine of the University of Warsaw helped by donating the necessary equipment for examination and measurement. Autopsies were occasionally performed, when the unceasing pressures of work in the hospitals allowed.

The study began in February 1942, but was broken off in the following summer simply because many physicians and others involved had been murdered. Many of the researchers were aware of their impending end. The transports from Warsaw to Treblinka began on 22 July, 1942. Adam Czerniakow, the head of the *Judenrat*, took his own life the next day. Until the middle of September – within seven weeks – some 300,000 Jews from the Warsaw Ghetto had been murdered in the gas chambers. The first commander of Treblinka, Dr. Imfried Eberl was the former director of the T4 institute in Brandenburg.

Several of the Jewish physicians in the ghetto were saved because of their profession. Some of them were transferred to augment the medical services in the Lodz Ghetto. The participants in the study who were not so lucky managed to hold discussions on its results before their transport to Treblinka. This was done under the auspices of the *Judenrat*, as noted in the prologue, and Dr. Milejkowski tried to secure their findings. A considerable part of the material was smuggled out of the ghetto into the Aryan part of Warsaw, and was entrusted to Dr. Wietold Orlowski of the faculty of medicine, one of Prof. Loth's nearest aides.

This material, originally written in Polish, was rediscovered after the War and published in French. The publication was forgotten until the Jewish American nutrition expert, Prof. Myron Winick, reawakened interest in the findings and published an English translation in 1979. The study is still considered the most comprehensive research done on the effects and implications of malnutrition. Contemporary researchers, such as the Israeli expert, Shaul Shasha, have confirmed its findings using the latest research methodologies.

The hunger studies conducted in the Warsaw Ghetto, and the continued clandestine medical studies there, were possibly the greatest expression of the Jewish intellectual protest and defiance of the Nazi doctors' destructive intentions and the medicalization of the Holocaust.

As transports continued to Treblinka, Ludwig Stabholz and his medical colleagues continued to offer aid to the sick and wounded, even as the number of the needy patients was dwindling daily. In April 1943, on the eve of the Warsaw Ghetto uprising, Stabholz's benefactor, Prof. Eduard Loth, sneaked into the ghetto, extricated Stabholz, removed him in a wheelchair with his own hands to the Aryan side and placed him in a safehouse. Loth was able to provide him with forged documents to hide his Jewish identity, and to prove that he helped with the German war effort. In the summer of 1944, during the Polish rebellion in Warsaw, Prof. Loth perished in the fighting. Stabholz and his wife managed to join the Soviet forces on the other side of the Vistula River and participated in the final offensive against the Germans.

Some of the Jewish physicians in the ghetto continued in their duties even through the ghetto uprising. The story, which took place in the previous months, of the physician Janusz Korczak, the great author of children's literature and educator, who declined to be spared and faithfully accompanied the pupils of his children's orphanage to the gas chambers, is well known. The story of Dr. Anna Braude-Heller, however, who managed a children's hospital in the ghetto, is remarkable as well. She had lost her own son to disease in the 1920s, and habitually walked about in black. Her bereavement made her even more devoted to the welfare of children. The hospital she ran was known for its high standards, though its state continuously deteriorated with the worsening conditions of the ghetto. The overcrowding reached the point where two or even three children were crammed into each bed. In the absence of medications, blankets and sufficient food, very little could be done to help these miserable children. The *Judenrat* provided the children's hospital with some milk and bread, but part of these provisions was taken by the hospital staff, themselves suffering from starvation. According to the data of the ghetto researcher, the physician Charles Roland, in the last quarter of 1941, the mortality rate in the children's hospital reached 24%. With the transports to Treblinka in summer 1942, the hospital was shut down altogether. According to the testimony of Adina Szwajger, a surviving member of the medical personnel, some of the children were given lethal injections – to spare them the suffering of death in the gas chambers. When the SS soldiers broke into the building, they shot the remaining children in their beds.

Dr. Anna Braude-Heller could have saved herself by being smuggled over to the Aryan side through her good connections with the Polish underground. This possibility was offered to her, as it was to Janusz Korczak – but she refused, and chose to remain in the ghetto together with the seventy thousand Jews who survived the massive wave of transports to Treblinka. She helped reorganize the medical services in the ghetto and worked in one of the remaining, functioning branches of Czyste Hospital. Anna's courage never left her. With the outbreak of the Warsaw Ghetto uprising in April, she stayed and kept administering to the wounded, until she perished in one of the bunkers, together with the last defenders of what had once been Europe's largest Jewish community.

Further reading

Götz Aly. **"Endlösung"; Völkersverschiebung und der Mord an den europäische Juden**. Frankfurt am Main: S. Fischer, 1995.

Christopher Browning. **Fateful Months: Essays on the Launching of the Final Solution.** New York: Cambridge University Press, 1992.

Nava Cohen. **Medicine in the Service of Ideology in the Third Reich: Its Role in the Anti-Jewish Policy in the Ghettos and Concentration Camps** (Hebrew). PhD Thesis submitted to the Hebrew University of Jerusalem. Jerusalem, 2002.

Charles G. Roland. **Courage under Siege; Starvation and Death in the Warsaw Ghetto.** New York: Oxford University Press, 1992.

Paul Weindling. **Epidemics and genocide in eastern Europe, 1890-1945.** New York: Oxford University Press, 2000.

Myron Winick (ed.). **Hunger Disease: Studies by the Jewish Physicians in the Warsaw Ghetto.** New York: John Wiley and Sons, 1979.

Chapter 8

Lodz Ghetto

Lodz, Poland's second largest city, was annexed to the German Reich after the conquest of Poland, by virtue of its large number of local inhabitants of German descent (*Volksdeutsche*). Its name was accordingly changed in April 1940 to Litzmannstadt, in honor of Karl Litzmann, the right-wing German general who captured it in World War I. A considerable portion of the city's non-German inhabitants – Poles and Jews – was expelled. After a period of time, some of the Jews were allowed to return – but under conditions of virtual slavery – as prisoners of a ghetto which the Nazis regarded as temporary. Their real intention was that "the ghetto and with it all the city of Lodz will be purged of Jews. The final goal *(Endziel)* must be to bring about the cauterization of this pestilential abscess" – as Nazi Governor Friedrich Übelhör, in his proposal to set up the Lodz Ghetto (December 1939), expressed it, using medical metaphors.

Lodz Ghetto was the second largest ghetto in all of Poland after Warsaw. At its height, about 200,000 Jews were crammed into it. It operated from April 1940 until the end of the war, in an old and poor section of the city. The sanitary conditions in the ghetto were terrible. Whole families, and even complete strangers, were crowded into a single room. Water, leaking into the decrepit old wooden houses, turned to ice in winter. The chilly rooms open to draughts were a constant source of respiratory illness. Firewood was rarely available. The general distress was exacerbated by a scarcity in clothing and shoes: all fur coats were confiscated by the Germans already in the winter of 1940-41. Additionally there was a chronic shortage of food, inadequate clean water, and problems of health care.

The Lodz Ghetto had, however, a certain distinction. The Jews of Lodz, numbering a full third of the city's population before the war, had historically pioneered the city's industrialization – notably the production of textiles, earning Lodz the title as "the Polish Manchester."

Of the city's factories, over a third were established and managed by Jews, as were a quarter of the smaller workshops. In addition, a large proportion of the Jewish heads of families earned their living as factory workers. The tradition of industrious, manual labor was well rooted among the Jews of Lodz, and many Jewish artisans were famous for the quality of their products.

With the establishment of the Lodz Ghetto, the Nazis decided to turn it into a center of production for the manufacture of the many goods wartime Germany needed, at home and for its armed forces. German entrepreneurs, like Hans Biebow, presented practical proposals to this effect, hoping to enrich themselves in the process. However it was Chaim Rumkowski, appointed by the Nazis to head the *Judenrat*, who realized the scheme. An authoritative, harsh and domineering man, Rumkowski was, nonetheless, a capable organizer, showing great zeal in persuading the Jews that their work for the Germans was their only chance to stay alive. He was firm in his belief that the key for survival of the ghetto Jews was in making them economically indispensable to the Germans. Rumkowski and the *Judenrat* under him were granted a semi-autonomous status by the Germans, including the authority to print postage stamps and currency bearing his image, meant strictly for ghetto use.

Rumkowski, who saw himself as the saviour of the ghetto, sought to leave a monument to himself and his deeds in the form of an orderly record. He employed an entire team of intellectuals and writers, most of them professional journalists, in order to precisely document all daily occurrences. Since the ghetto chronicle was open for German inspection, it could not always describe faithfully the details of the horrors taking place. However, thanks to this chronicle, we have a wealth of information about the conditions of health and medicine in Lodz Ghetto. Other testimonies and secondary historical literature, such as Michal Unger's comprehensive book in Hebrew (2005), were used to complete the description.

The Ghetto health department

The extensive *Judenrat* organization of the Lodz Ghetto included a sizable health department. In the summer of 1942, it numbered about two thousand workers, including two hundred physicians. During 1941, the number of physicians doubled with the transfer of a hundred or so doctors from Warsaw and Central Europe. The justification for this was the necessity of preserving the health of the productive population, to ensure they would be able to continue working and producing for the Germans. This logic dictated that Jews who were ill should be treated quickly and returned to work as fast as possible. Their families, including children, were considered – at least by the *Judenrat* and the health department – also worthy of medical treatment, as a contribution to maintaining morale and as partial compensation for the meager pay allotted to the Jewish forced laborers.

For a time, the Germans assented to this arrangement. As a result, until the autumn of 1942 the ghetto had a well-functioning medical system, including a few large hospitals and many clinics. The largest hospital, on Lagiewnicka Street, housed many different wards: internal, surgical, gynecological, ophthalmic, pediatric and more, and had some four hundred beds. In addition, a maternity hospital of three hundred beds operated in

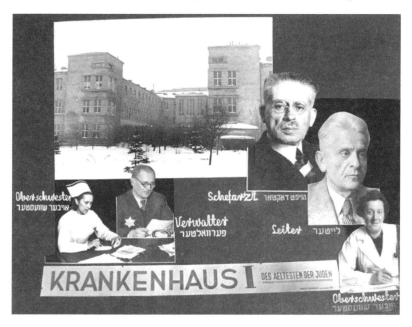

Lodz ghetto largest hospital with some personnel. Courtesy of Yad Vashem Archives.

the first two years of the ghetto, and also a hospital for infectious diseases, in which sophisticated laboratory tests were carried out.

Medical research was also carried out in the ghetto, though on a smaller scale than in Warsaw and mostly by individual physicians. Not surprisingly, the emphasis was on subjects connected with nutrition. Thus a study was carried out on growth disturbances among adolescents as a result of undernourishment. Another study was undertaken by a veterinary doctor, and dealt with the quality of horsemeat which served as an important source of protein in the ghetto. In the absence of motor vehicles, horses were used for transportation. A special carriage was adapted as a makeshift ambulance for patients, which was drawn by horses. The horses often succumbed to the hardship (their food was also limited), and their flesh was used as food.

The day-to-day medical and hygienic activity in the ghetto was managed by the health department of the *Judenrat*, under the medical direction of Dr. Leon Szykier. The administrative director was Jozef Rumkowski – brother of the *Judenrat* chairman. This arrangement proved untenable for Dr. Szykier, who was forced to resign in May 1941. Dr. Viktor Miller was appointed in his place, and continued in this post until the liquidation of the ghetto. A medical council of sorts existed in the ghetto, as a framework for physician in-service training, headed by a woman, Dr. Klausenberg. Other women also held responsible posts, such as Dr. Sima Mandels, who headed the child care section, and Dr. Jokisz-Grinberg, one of the chiefs of the health department.

In its prime, the health department controlled an impressive network of seven hospitals, five clinics, seven pharmacies, two emergency stations, two preventive clinics and two nursing homes for the elderly. Gradually other tasks were added as well: school sanitation services, a department of preventive hygiene, and even an institute for the testing of foodstuff and veterinary inspection.

A number of other factors contributed to improved hygienic conditions and the provision of quality preventive medicine. The TOZ organisation was active in Lodz, and provided inoculations for children. Specialists practiced dentistry and pharmacology, paid by private patients. In July 1941, a sanatorium was opened in Marysin, outside the ghetto, which served mainly those favoured by the *Judenrat*. Marysin was also the site of the city cemetery, which was increasingly used by the ghetto Jews.

Between 1940 and 1942, the number of dead in the ghetto rose threefold or even fourfold.

For a lengthy period, the Germans were unwilling to intervene in the ghetto health arrangements. Only one unique event was recorded in the chronicles. In July 1941, a German committee of race experts entered the ghetto to study the medical histories of hospitalized psychiatric patients. Careful records were made, and some weeks afterwards, two German physicians arrived to organize the transport of these patients to extermination camps.

The *Judenrat* made attempts to improve the poor diet in the ghetto. The Germans portioned out a much greater amount of food than in Warsaw – about 1,400 calories a day per capita – but this was still insufficient. Furthermore, food distribution suffered from great inconstancy. Lodz was located in an isolated area, cut off from the rest of Poland, making the smuggling of food very difficult.

The *Judenrat* set up public kitchens and dining rooms, mostly near the factories. An attempt was made, not always successfully, to have special supplemental rations granted for the benefit of the workers, so that at least the productive workers would be able to receive an additional serving of soup and one more slice of bread per day.

The ghetto inhabitants suffered from a constant state of hunger, or at least of undernourishment, severely affecting their health. In particular, the lack of proteins and fats was evident. Oskar Rozenfeld, one of the chroniclers, described the plight of the ghetto Jews as "a lingering dying." The situation had its inevitable influence on the productivity of laborers in the workshops. At times workers, under unremitting pressure by their supervisors to increase the quotas of production, simply collapsed from weakness. The chronicle reports that on a single day, January 5, 1942, no fewer than 172 workers fainted at their machines. Presumably, the freezing conditions of that winter day contributed to this.

The workers did not permit themselves to be absent from work for more than a few days, fearing dismissal. In addition, absence from work also meant the relinquishing of the additional food provided only in the factories. Finally, a lessening production could weaken the German determination to preserve the ghetto. The *Judenrat* tried, therefore, to improvise new means for improvement of nourishment, such as the growing of vegetables, potatoes in particular, within the ghetto and also outside, in an attempt to overcome the severe vitamin deficiency. Even the grounds of the cemetery at Marysin were put to use for this purpose.

Morbidity in the Ghetto and the collapse of the hospitalization

Despite all efforts, mortality rates continued to climb relentlessly. In the summer of 1942, the death rate reached two percent of the population per month – ten times that for Lodz before the war. The rate of mortality was as high as that of Warsaw Ghetto. The chief causes of death in the years 1941-42 were tuberculosis and the severe malnutrition. Deaths from starvation were often disguised, for the benefit of the authorities, as being from other causes, notably heart disease.

In the autumn of 1942, the living situation of the ghetto Jews worsened dramatically. The Germans had made a drastic decision to reduce the ghetto population, by getting rid of anyone who was not a productive worker, and therefore considered expendable. Probably the mass deportation at the same time of Jews from Warsaw to the death camp in Treblinka had some connection with this decision.

The most malevolent decree was aimed at the children of Lodz Ghetto. The Nazis ordered the murder of all children under ten. Rumkowski, himself childless, fought to save at least the ten-year-olds, who, he argued, were capable of working. After this, he bravely went out and stood before the Jews of the ghetto, asking them to willingly surrender their children, elderly and ill to the Germans. He told them on September 4, 1942:

> I must stretch out my hands and beg: brothers and sisters, hand them over to me […]. Fathers and mothers: give me your children […]. I must cut off limbs, in order to save the body! I must take children, and if not, others may – God forbid! – be taken…

Rumkowski called this Nazi plan "a diabolic plot," describing himself as "a bandit" who has come "to take away the dearest": but his logic was that of some Jewish physicians in Auschwitz who later faced a similar terrible impasse, compelled to make the selection of those to be sent to their deaths. "Common sense dictates that those to be saved are those who have the best chances of survival, and not those who do not by any means have the possibility of being saved."

Few complied with Rumkowski's impossible plea. As a consequence, in the beginning of September, the Nazis unleashed a raid of hitherto-unknown proportions. They announced a curfew, invaded the streets and houses in the ghetto and tore children and old people from the arms of their families. Many were murdered on the spot; the streets flowed with blood. The remainder, nearly 20,000 children and old people, were sent to the newly-established extermination camp in Chelmno.

These scenes of horror occurred also in the hospitals. All hospitals were liquidated along with their patients. At dawn on the first of September, 1,700 patients and a portion of the medical staff were dragged out and dispatched to Chelmno. Some were shot trying to escape. One of the hospitals was set on fire. Any relatives refusing to part from the patients were compelled to accompany them to extermination. Even the generally restrained language of the chronicle gives a poignant description of what was happening:

> How much toil and trouble was involved in being admitted to the hospital? What special privilege was needed to obtain a bed, even in the corridor, in the passageway? How happy was the family who was able to commit its dear one to treatment in the hospital! [...] And here, suddenly – the tragedy of the patients and their families is indescribable. One has a brother, a second has a sister, this one a father, that one a mother, cousin, aunt! Everyone left someone. [Such] scenes of horror were not yet seen [...] weeping and wailing [...]. In the case of children's diseases, the patients were kept on purpose longer in the hospital, in order to prevent the spread of epidemics. And here these children, who actually became healthy, became victims of this terrible order [...]. Out of fear of having his old mother sent, the son died from a heart attack, and the mother who was a candidate for hospitalization was taken by the Jewish police [faithful accomplices for the transports – D.N.] two hours later. Another woman escaped in fright from the hospital the day after she gave birth, and today she died.

Many managed to escape from the hospitals in spite of their poor physical condition. Some of them were convalescents who stayed in

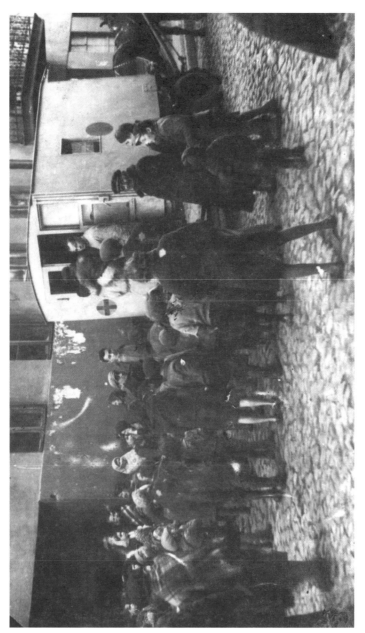

A horse drawn "ambulance" in the Lodz ghetto. Courtesy of Yad Vashem Archives.

the hospital by virtue of some favor (or bribe) and thereby enjoyed an improved diet. In the days following, the Germans demanded that the *Judenrat* hand over all escapees. When the order was not obeyed, escapees' family members were taken into custody.

The new pattern of Ghetto health services

Following an outbreak of typhoid fever, the contagious diseases hospital was reopened; the Germans constantly feared the spread of such diseases to their own camp.

The rest of the medical system changed its nature: the emphasis shifted to offering treatment in the workshops and factories. All survivors, including children of ten years and upwards, were now working in the workshops of the different manufacture branches (which were now called "*Ressorts*"). Small and large clinics were maintained there, according to the size of the *Ressort*. Each large factory, employing over a thousand workers had at least one full-time *Ressort* physician.

A new medical arrangement was instituted: a system of district medical services. Within the ghetto, forty districts were delineated, each under the supervision of at least one family doctor. Each such physician was meant to provide treatment to some 1000-2500 people. These district doctors received patients in infirmaries, but occasionally paid house calls. Two expert clinics were maintained and a first-aid service, with two treatment stations, to which the ill and injured were brought in horse-drawn carts.

The most prevalent disease in the ghetto was tuberculosis, which infected about half the ghetto population and caused the deaths of over ten thousand patients. Illnesses of the alimentary tract were also prevalent. In the summer of 1941, a dysentery epidemic wiped out about two-thirds of all babies within few months. Many others suffered from typhoid fever and spotted typhus.

Intestinal illnesses were such a problem that the chronicles tried to list the reasons for them. The chronicle of September 25, 1942, mentions one of the main reasons:

Among the infectious diseases, the most frequent is typhoid fever. In certain houses, one can count the number of flats containing typhoid patients, because of the crowding, isolation is unthinkable [...]

that is why this disease increases and spreads in an ever-widening circle. [In addition] they live in filth, sleep in filth, and also eat without keeping basic hygienic conditions. The vegetables [good quantities of vegetables were grown in the ghetto itself – D.N.] are not properly washed. There is no warm water for washing, and no time to deal with this and also prepare meals […]. Nobody waits for the food to be properly cooked, and when everyone is hungry, they swallow half-cooked food, which is, in most cases, the cause of the illness […]. And if we add to these conditions the absolute lack recently of all sorts of medications, like tenalbin, opium, and other means against diarrhea, it is easy to understand how terrible is the situation. And so, from simple reasons, even light illnesses sometimes end up in death.

Sometime after this was written the conditions of patients of intestinal disorders and other diseases improved, with the renewed opening of hospitals in the ghetto. For the next two years, with the reorganization of the health system, a real improvement in medical statistics was noted.

The last days of the ghetto

The ghetto mortality rate in the years 1943-44 stabilized at a much lower rate than in previous years. The health department was successful in combating and halting the typhus epidemics which broke out in 1943. One of the explanations for this improvement was the simple fact that the remaining ghetto population, about 100,000, no longer included small children, elderly people and the chronically ill, most of whom had been dispatched to the gas chambers in the horrible events of September 1942. A relatively easier, more stable period followed, lasting a further two years. Improvements were registered in food rations for the productive population, which consisted mainly of young men and women – especially soup, which contained chiefly potatoes and other vegetables.

Occasionally the Germans granted the *Judenrat* permission to buy medications – at full market value – from the income earned by the ghetto industries, lucrative production for which Hans Biebow paid very little. He and the German administrators he bribed had an interest in preserving the work force that was accruing such enormous profits for them. It looked like Rumkowski's dream of preserving the productive part of the ghetto was about to be realized. However, the advance of the Soviet Army towards the region in the spring of 1944 was the harbinger of the end of the ghetto, since named "the last ghetto."[1] The Germans began dismantling the factories and sent the valuable equipment back to Germany. The Jewish workers, however, were destined for extermination.

By the end of June 1944, the transfer of thousands of Jews from the ghetto to the death camp at Chelmno had begun, reopened especially for this purpose. In August, tens of thousands more were sent to Auschwitz. In this period, there was a renewed weakening of health and medical care. Even the physicians lost all hope, on the brink of the catastrophe, and no longer had the strength to combat the various illnesses. Again, the most destructive disease was tuberculosis, causing the death of over five hundred patients in one month, July 1944.

Only eight hundred Jews, still needed by the Germans, managed to survive in Lodz, until its liberation by the Russians in January 1945. Several of them, including the physician Daniel Weisskopf, hid in bunkers – but a short time before the Russian arrival, Biebow and his henchmen discovered their hiding place. Dr. Weisskopf along with his bunker companions were shot in cold blood.

Further reading

The Chronicle of the Lodz Ghetto, 1941-1944 (ed. by Lucian Dubroszycki). New Haven, Conn.: Yale University Press, 1984. [A complete German translation appeared recently. Göttingen: Wallstein Verlag, 2007. 5 Vols.].
Isajah Trunk. **Lodz Ghetto; A History.** Bloomington, Ind.: Indiana University Press, 2006.

---

1   This is also the title of Michal Unger's book mentioned before (Jerusalem: Yad Vashem, 2005).

Chapter 9

Šiauliai and Kaunas Ghettos and Partisan Doctors

Jewish physicians were active in all ghettos, large and small. In one of the smaller ghettos a unique testimony has been left of such activities, which provides a valuable personal insight into the harrowing dilemmas confronting the physicians. It is a testimony to their having to wrestle with their consciences in fulfilling nearly impossible duties. A diary was written during those hard times – a uniquely human and beautifully written document testifying to the difficulties he experienced – left by the physician, Aharon Pick, of the Šiauliai Ghetto in Lithuania.

Šiauliai ghetto

Before the war, the city of Šiauliai in northern Lithuania was home to about 5,400 Jews. Several hundred Jewish refugees were added to the community following the division of Poland in 1939 between Germany and the Soviet Union. In June 1941, about a thousand members of the community managed to escape to Russia a few days before Šiauliai fell to the Germans on June 26, 1941. The Germans and Lithuanians murdered another thousand Jews in the first two weeks of the occupation. At the end of July, a ghetto was enclosed in the city, into which many of the Jews of neighboring towns were also crowded. A *Judenrat* of five members was appointed, chaired by Mendel Leibowicz.

Before the occupation, the Jewish community had a small hospital of forty beds. Since the location of this hospital was outside the ghetto, a substitute was found, with a unique location – the Jewish cemetery, in what had been the charnel house and caretakers' lodgings. These makeshift quarters served for cures, treatments, births and even surgery, performed by an anti-Semitic Lithuanian surgeon who, having been paid a large sum of money, was willing to temporarily suspend his animosity towards Jews. This so-called hospital was most poorly provided for, lacking any X-ray equipment for instance.

Dr. Aharon pick and his diary

Dr. Aharon Pick, the writer of the diary documenting events in the Ghetto, was a man of many interests. He was born in 1872 in Kaidan, near Kaunas, the second largest city in Lithuania. A precocious child, he was destined to become a rabbi, and studied in a rabbinical seminary in Kaunas, but was also drawn to secular studies. For a time he served as a Hebrew teacher in a school, before setting out for Paris to study medicine. After World War I, having worked as a physician in Paris and specializing in radiology, he returned to Lithuania, settling in Šiauliai, where he directed the department of internal medicine in the local hospital. In addition, he had a private practice and was one of the founders of the Hebrew secondary school in the city. Pick also

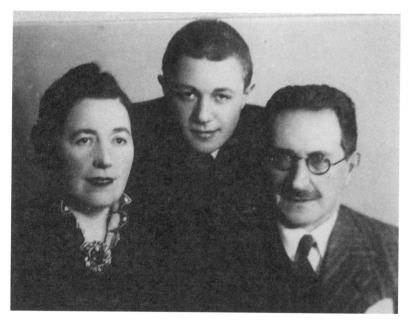

Dr. Aharon Pick, his wife Deborah and their son David. Courtesy of Mrs. Chaya Pick.

served as head of the local branch of the Association for Preserving the Health among the Jews, OZA, and supervised the health of the city's Jewish school children. His home was the meeting-place for the city's intelligentsia, and a center of Zionist activity.

In 1936, he traveled to Paris in order to observe the medical advances displayed in the World Fair. On the train journey through Nazi Germany, he happened to buy the Nazi newspaper, **Der Stürmer**. He was shocked by its vicious anti-Semitic contents, but could not imagine the storm to be unleashed in the years ahead.

When the Nazis overran Lithuania, Dr. Pick was already sixty-eight years old and due to retire from his position in the hospital. He was ready to become a pensioner and enjoy the leisure of a well-respected public man, who could look back on his life's work with satisfaction. Instead, he was fated to witness the horrors of the Holocaust in his city. Even in the early stages of the Nazi conquest, he took it upon himself to document all happenings, while continuing his medical work. Though multilingual, he chose to write his diary in, of all languages, Hebrew – perhaps as a Jewish act of defiance against the Nazis, or perhaps he thought that this would help preserve his writings from being read by hostile eyes. He kept on writing whenever he could find spare time, filling three thick notebooks bound in cardboard. He gave his diary a most suitable name: **Notes from the Valley of Death**.

While recording events, he continued his heavy schedule of medical duties in a clinic separate from the hospital, specializing in radiology. Though fully aware of the deplorable state of the ghetto hospital, he refused the offer to become its manager. He was not willing to bear the responsibility for the draconian measures needed in order to comply with the demands of the Nazis.

Dr. Pick kept up his writing until his last days in the Šiauliai Ghetto in the summer of 1944. He died a short time before the liberation of the city by the Red Army, of natural causes, for he was already seventy-two years old. It seems certain that the difficult circumstances aided in the decline of his health. His last entry in his journal bore the date of the seventh of June 1944 – a day after the start of the Allied invasion of Normandy. This knowledge might have comforted him in his last days. He was also spared the sight of the final liquidation of the ghetto, about a month after his death. He could still be buried with dignity in the final days of the ghetto.

Dr. Pick's son, David, hid his father's diaries in a sealed tin container, depositing them in a safe place before fleeing for his life. After the Russian conquest of Lithuania, some relatives retrieved the diary and smuggled it into Israel where it was kept in private hands for years. The fearful owner hesitated to publish it because of the several harsh descriptions it contained. Eventually, a young scholar, Miriam Offer, rediscovered the papers and it was published in 1998 by the Association of former Lithuanian Jews. Dr. Aharon Pick's diary, written in excellent literary Hebrew, is the principal source of the history of the Šiauliai ghetto and the account of the medical services provided by the Jewish physicians in the face of the Nazi dictatorial inhuman orders.

Jewish doctors' dilemmas

Dr. Pick's diary records the harsh medical decrees imposed upon the ghetto by the Nazis, orders Dr. Pick and his colleagues not only had to obey, but were forced to become accomplices in their enforcement. One such order forbade the transfer of patients with infectious diseases to the local hospital:

> The injunction coincided with the epidemic of spotted typhus, which has begun spreading in Lithuania, and reached Šiauliai. It was patently known to our rulers, that in the ghetto […] there is no place of refuge for those ill with infectious diseases. The epidemic caused terrible dread for all in the ghetto, who are largely inflicted with the lice, teeming in the crowded and filthy dwellings, which are, as is well known, the Angels of Death of this disease. We will not be guilty of exaggeration or sin against the truth if we assume that this decree has been issued with deliberate forethought to endanger the ghetto, with a design for the disease to spread throughout its entirety, so there would be an excellent excuse to liquidate the whole ghetto in one stroke.

In this description we can see, in a different guise, the medicalization of the Holocaust, already evidenced in the Warsaw Ghetto. Dr. Pick was not naïve, and he continued questioning: "This excuse, what purpose does it serve? And why is it at all needed? Is there a necessity for any excuse when they desire to exterminate some thousands of Jews? A slight hint will be enough and the execution will be carried out with a decisive exactness." He foresaw, unfortunately, the inevitable end of the ghetto.

We also learn from the diary of the order forbidding the obtaining of medications at the local pharmacies in the city. The inhabitants found a solution by opening a pharmacy within the ghetto, with a chemical laboratory of sorts, where substitutes for medicaments and unavailable health products, such as toothpaste, were prepared. The emphasis was on the concoction of compounds and preparations from plants and herbs.

The most severe decree was issued to the ghetto on the fifth of February 1942: the local *Judenrat* was ordered to prevent births in the ghetto. This of course was part of what Dr. Marc Dvorjetski has called "the biological warfare"[1] which the Nazis committed against the Jewish and other "inferior" people. Dr. Pick recorded in his diary: "The day our representatives were given this decree, humiliating us to the level of beasts, must remain in memory for eternity." He could not withhold his further comment: "What is only lacking is the castration of the men and women, and then the decree might be carried out to its full end."

The *Judenrat* was charged with bringing this injunction to everyone's knowledge. The announcement caused a great shock to all the Jews in the ghetto. The public was warned: "Births in the ghetto are unwanted. Most severe means will be carried out against Jewish women giving birth. Artificial abortions will not be prosecuted." A six month period of extension was granted to women in the fourth month of pregnancy and beyond. A month before the end of the extended deadline, the chief of the German security police in Šiauliai fixed August 15, 1942 as the final date for permissible births. If it would become known that any birth has occurred after this date, the child, the mother and her entire family would be put to death, and the *Judenrat* leaders would bear personal responsibility.

The ghetto representatives were forced to warn the public: "Time passes. The final hour [...] is not far. Remember, Jewish women, that after the 15th of August there will be no more births in the ghetto hospital [...]

---

1   This was the title of one of Dvorjetski's books, published in 1959. Marc Dvorjetski will be dealt with in more detail in the next chapter.

and births in private houses are likewise forbidden." Physicians, midwives and all other persons were forbidden to assist Jewish women in giving birth. Anyone transgressing this order would suffer severe punishment. Pick wrote in his diary: "This wicked decree has never been heard at all throughout history, and will not ever be forgotten; how can one's heart not burst to hear of such things?"

The *Judenrat* and ghetto physicians held frequent consultations on how to deal with this evil. It was clear that some women would not be willing to obey the order and would insist on giving birth in spite of all warnings. Their intransigence could spell danger not only to the mothers and their families, but also to the entire ghetto. Measures were decided upon to deal with potential disobedience of these dire orders, from the denial of medical aid for the mother – in the thought that this may lead indirectly to the death of the baby – through the punishment of the whole family by denial of food, to the last resort – putting the child to death.

The director of the ghetto hospital, Dr. Wolf Pesachowicz, and the chief physician, Dr. Burstein (appointed because of his knowledge of German), expressed their clear preference for the severer approach. They probably feared for their own lives if they would show any signs of opposition to the inhuman decrees forced upon the ghetto.

Dr. Pick gave full expression to the feelings of frustration and disgust about the predicament, since he was eventually and unwillingly forced to be active in the killing of some newborn babies. On December 10, 1943, he recorded in his journal: "Certain details in our cursed life will never be erased from our memories. It is utterly unbelievable that we, cultured men of conscience and high principles, have descended catastrophically to such low, that we have been made into killers and murderers." He further described in his diary what happened in the ghetto following the Nazi orders:

The evil decree forbidding births in the ghetto still stands in force. In spite of the dangers overtaking the entire ghetto over such occurrences, some births have taken place anyway, and normal children have been born, by dint of the women who refused to end their pregnancies in time. It is incumbent on us, the physicians, to put the living, healthy and normal children to death, in order to extricate the entire ghetto

from the danger of perdition and oblivion. And it is we who must
execute this heinous and ignoble mission...

The rest of the entry describes the horrifying details of the way
children's lives were ended. They refused to die even after having been
systematically starved and denied milk or water.

Dr. Pick's scientific character wondered about the will to live of a
tender baby, condemned to be put to death by the physicians in such a
cruel manner: "I would never have believed that a child who has just
seen the light of day will be so powerfully anchored to life. Such a trial
is not [to be found] in the literature, for who is it who would attempt to
starve a child for seven-eight consecutive days?"

The occurrences in the Šiauliai Ghetto were not unique, but we have
been bequeathed no record to parallel the detailed description and the
literary talent of Dr. Aharon Pick. The depth of horror in his descriptions
is what possibly prevented the publication of his diary for so many
years.

Kaunas (Kovno) Ghetto

The Chairman of the Kaunas Ghetto *Judenrat* was a physician,
Dr. Elchanan Elkes, a dignified and highly moral man, who tirelessly
tried to ease the lot of the Jews in the ghetto, numbering some 30,000
Jews in the summer of 1941. The leaders of the community found him
unanimously to be the most suitable candidate for the job and Elkes
accepted the difficult post with a heavy heart. Despite his age (he was 62)
and less-than-perfect health, he took upon himself the full responsibility,
which also included standing courageously before the Nazi persecutors
and striving to defend the interests of his people in the face of merciless
killers, confronting them boldly while knowingly endangering his own
safety. He bravely refused to accede to any order to the *Judenrat* to hand
over even a single Jew for extermination. On the contrary – he tried his
best to save from death Jews caught in different raids. On October 28,
1941, during one of these desperate attempts, he was seriously wounded
by a Nazi policeman and was saved by emergency treatment from his
fellow doctors in a nearby house. It took a few days until he was out of
danger and could be brought back to his own home.

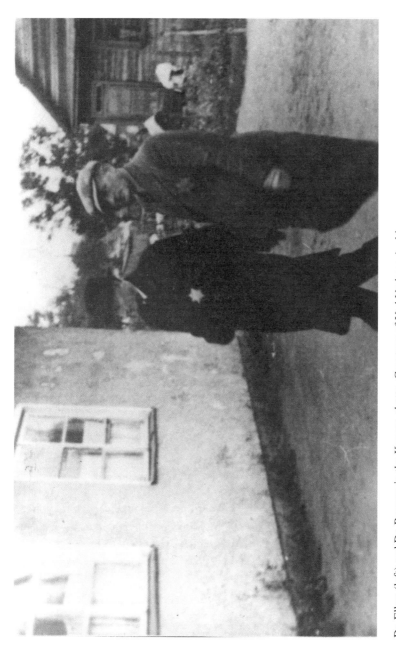

Dr. Elkes (left) and Dr. Berman in the Kaunas ghetto. Courtesy of Yad Vashem Archives.

As head of the *Judenrat,* Dr. Elkes was highly regarded by all because of his character and devotion, and even the Germans came to respect his honesty and discretion. He did much to maintain and even expand the ghetto medical services, which included a new hospital inaugurated towards the end of 1941. The previous one had been burned down by the Germans. Head of the hospital was Dr. Elkes' trusted aide, Dr. Moshe Berman. Immediately following their occupation of Kaunas, towards the end of June 1941, the Germans slaughtered thousands of Jews. The next two-and-a-half years were relatively quiet, however. Most adults were put to work for the German army. Workshops were set up, and forced labor parties were sent out during the day to military installations outside the ghetto. The only wages for their work were food rations, which of course were far from sufficient. The ghetto health services strove to mitigate the effects of deficient nourishment and to halt the increasing morbidity.

In the winter of 1942, as in the Šiauliai Ghetto, the Germans issued a prohibition against all Jewish births in the Kaunas Ghetto. They charged the *Judenrat* with enforcing this inhuman decree and conducting a campaign against pregnancies.

From the winter of 1944, the persecution of the Jews in the Kaunas Ghetto intensified. Dr. Elkes did all he could to soften the impact of the worst orders. An underground Jewish resistance operated in the ghetto, and Dr. Elkes offered it all the support he could, supplying funds to purchase and manufacture weapons, and helping members to escape and continue the struggle against the Germans as partisans.

In March 1944, nearly two thousand old people, women and children were murdered. In June the Germans began transferring the remnants of the ghetto to concentration camps and forced labor sites in Germany. Elkes himself was sent to the Landsberg camp near Munich, where he was placed in charge of the camp sickroom. Having refused to participate in selections for extermination of those considered unfit, he went on a hunger strike and died of illness on October 1944, a proud man of principle and integrity to the end.

Armed resistance of Jewish physicians against the Nazis

In several ghettos, Jewish physicians took an active role in the armed resistance against their German oppressors. In one of the first uprisings, in the Lachva Ghetto in Belarus, Dr. Igelnick was a full participant in the revolt, which broke out in early September 1942. Some of the inhabitants of the ghetto broke through the fences and fled to the forests. There they joined the partisans and carried on guerrilla resistance against the Germans. The Lachva Ghetto fighters inflicted casualties on the Germans, and Dr. Igelnick refused to treat those German soldiers wounded while suppressing the insurrection. In response, he was shot to death on the spot.

A well-known case of a physician who led the struggle against the Germans in Belarus is that of Dr. Yekhezkiel Atlas, a young doctor who commanded a Jewish partisan unit of several dozen ghetto-escapees-turned-fighters, including some medical personnel and even a couple of dentists. These partisans protected the Jewish families who found refuge in the woods. They also launched reprisals against the Germans in revenge for the massacre of the Jews of Dereczyn (July 1942), proving their daring and bravery. Dr. Atlas, who became famous as a dauntless and resourceful fighter, met his death in battle on December 1942. In 1964 Samuel Bornstein published a book (in Hebrew) commemorating him and his band of Jewish fighters.

A particularly interesting story is that of Dr. Abraham Blumowicz, who was active in the armed underground of the Slonim Ghetto in Belarus. In the spring of 1942, he escaped to the forests with his personal weapons, guaranteeing his inclusion in a band of partisans, who were generally reluctant to accept Jews into their ranks. Unfortunately, he had not escaped with his medical equipment, forcing him to improvise makeshift medical instruments from available tools, like chisels, wherever he found them, and with these primitive devices he treated his wounded partisan comrades, and even performed successful surgery. According to the testimony of surviving partisans, he was able to save the lives of many fighters.

After the Red Army had liberated the area, Blumowicz was placed at the head of a large Russian military hospital in the Brest-Litovsk area, which treated many thousands of soldiers. After the war, he and his family remained for two years in a Jewish refugee camp near Munich, where he was active in the leadership of the displaced persons after the Holocaust. David Ben-Gurion, the future first prime minister of the State of Israel, met him there in 1946. Upon hearing he was a physician, and greatly impressed with his experience, Ben-Gurion urged him to immigrate to Palestine and join the emerging Jewish army medical services.

Blumowicz arrived two years later, in June 1948, and upon Ben-Gurion's intercession (who also suggested that he change his foreign-sounding family name to the Hebrew name of "Atzmon"), was appointed chief medical officer for the northern front in the decisive phase of Israel's War of Independence. In February 1949, Atzmon was promoted to serve as the Israeli army chief medical officer, the second to hold that post, with the rank of *sgan aluf* (colonel). He worked to instill a sense of greater professionalism and discipline in the Israeli medical corps, holding the position at its head until September 1956.

Further reading

Anthology of Holocaust Literature (ed. by J. Glatstein and others). Philadelphia: Jewish Publication Society of America, 1949. pp. 299 ff.

Aharon Pick. **Notes from the Valley of Death** (Hebrew). Tel Aviv: Association of Former Lithuanian Jews, 1998.

Avraham Tory. **Surviving the Holocaust; the Kovno Ghetto Diary.** Cambridge, Mass.: Harvard University Press, 1990.

Chapter 10

Marc Dvorjetski – a Doctor in the Ghettos and Labor Camps

Dr. Marc Dvorjetski's memories of his experiences during the Holocaust are unquestionably of great value. He personally experienced the atrocities of the period as a Jew and a physician. Then, on coming to Israel after the war, he pioneered the study of the medical aspects of the Holocaust.

In **Bein Habtarim**, his memoirs published in 1956 in Hebrew, Dr. Dvorjetski related his experiences during the Holocaust. He regarded his writings almost as an expiation of sorts, the apology of a survivor, and an affirmation of humanity in the face of bestial inhumanity. He openly wondered about the reason for his own survival, and wrestled with his sense of guilt. Had he perhaps committed a sin by remaining alive, when millions of others, no less worthy than himself, perished. His conscience condemned him with the thoughts:

> "What did you do to deserve the 'certificate of life'? Perhaps you were false to me – my Conscience – while being tortured, or by being confronted with temptation in the ghetto and the concentration camps? Perhaps you sold me for the price of staying alive? Were you not also among those in the ghettos and camps, who redeemed themselves at the expense of their brothers?"

Dr. Dvorjetski emerged from these inner questionings assured of his innocence, and was able to reply to his conscience:

> "It seems that I am capable of looking you in the eye, my Conscience; I did not sell you, and I surely did not betray you." He even provides some examples of this: "When the time came, and it was decreed that all those in Vilnius Ghetto would be put to death,

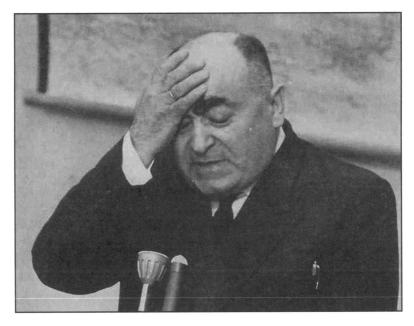

Dr. Marc Dvorjetski testifying at Eichmann's Trial (1961). Courtesy of Prof. Estee Dvorjetski.

save for those who possessed the yellow certificates, referred to as 'Life Certificates' – and their number was very much fewer than the number of people – and I won my Life Certificate by drawing lots with my friend, Dr. Kolodner… it was purely by Fate that I chanced to draw the possibility of life… and when I served as the section physician of the ghetto health services, it was demanded of me one day to draw up a list of old people in my quarter – and I guessed to what use this list may be put some day. I did not attempt at all to seek out old people in my quarter – and resigned from my position."

Dr. Dvorjetski continued recounting his experiences during the Holocaust:

"In the Vaivara concentration camp in Estonia, when the camp commander ordered me to be a work overseer, I answered that I am unable to serve in this position, since I am incapable of ordering others to work, and so I remained a cleaner of latrines, and some others were found who would order me around, hurry me at work and inspect me... And at the Stutthof camp, where we had to carry stretchers loaded with coal while running, and when I was told again to oversee the coal carriers (which meant being free of hard labor and receiving double rations of food), I preferred to be myself among the 'runners' who carried their heavy loads... rather than wield a club over my brothers' backs... 'Lead us not into temptation' – my thoughts tremble within me when I recall those who were led into temptation: their choice being either death, or to carry with their very hands the victims to the crematoria. My good fortune did not cause me to suffer such a choice... I withstood my small temptations, and did not sell you, my Conscience..."

Dr. Marc Dvorjetski served first in the ghetto of Vilnius, the city of his birth, where he had worked many years as a physician. The Vilnius Ghetto was opened in the beginning of September 1941. After a few raids in which around twenty thousand Jews were exterminated in the nearby Ponary Forest, about forty thousand still remained. Mass murder continued, however, and by the beginning of 1942 only some 24,000 remained, of whom two-thirds were put to work for the German war production. As in Lodz, the local Jewish Council (*Judenrat*) led by Jakob Gens believed that the Jews in the ghetto would not be killed if they remained useful as forced laborers for the German war effort. The ghetto maintained an active cultural life, including a well-known theater and library, and also a reasonably developed system of health services.

Dr. Dvorjetski worked for over a year in the ghetto's hospital. He noted the resourcefulness of some of his colleagues (while being modest about his own achievements). Some of the doctors were gifted with inventiveness, like Dr. Fingerhut of Warsaw, who managed to manufacture vitamins as a preventive remedy for severe skin infections threatening the ghetto children, or Dr. Lazar Finkelstein, who devised iodine products in order to successfully combat widespread goitre. All physicians toiled steadfastly to combat the spread of typhus, and labored twenty-four hours a day in the treatment of their patients. All the while, they were apprehensive that there may not be any sense in curing people who would simply be sent to their death that day or the next.

In addition to his medical work and the beginning of his documentation of ghetto life, Dr. Dvorjetski was active in the ghetto resistance movement. He instructed several nurses who intended to escape and join the partisans in the adjacent forests. He himself planned to escape to the forests, but the Germans surprised him first, and sent him and several other doctors to labor camps in Estonia.

Dr. Dvorjetski found himself in some of the most arduous camps in an area which had been purged of its Jewish population (*Judenrein*) at an earlier stage, but now contained tens of thousands of forced-labor Jewish prisoners transferred there from all conquered areas in the Soviet Union, the Baltic states and, from 1942, Theresienstadt, to be used as slave labor to exploit the natural resources of the area for the benefit of the German war effort. Twenty such labor camps existed in Estonia, the most important of which were manufacturing a fuel substitute from locally quarried bituminous shale.

On September 3, 1943, Dr. Dvorjetski himself arrived at the Vaivara camp, the largest and most central in Estonia – but for the next year and a half, he was shunted between five or six other camps in the area. Vaivara served as the administrative center of all Estonian camps, under the commandant *Obersturmbahnführer* Hans Aumeier, who previously served as commandant of Auschwitz. The chief physician of the camps was the SS *Sturmführer* Dr. Franz von Bothmann, whose cruel behavior towards Jewish prisoner-doctors was notorious. He physically assaulted Dr. Dvorjetski more than once. Bothmann took an active part in the occasional selections in the camps, in particular with regard to epidemics, which terrified the Germans and motivated draconian measures to fight them.

In some of the camps where there was no resident doctor, the Germans appointed an ordinary SS orderly in his place. Since the camps' central administration was instructed to reduce the death rate of slave workers, Jewish prisoner-doctors, known simply as "caretakers" (*Pfleger*), were charged with taking care of the prisoners to the best of their abilities. Some of the Jewish physicians were designated as "traveling caretakers." Their duty was to move about with the prisoner-workers and provide medical aid to those injured in work accidents or from the blows of overseers. Dr. Dvorjetski remarked that he doubted if such a title was part of the official standard of the camps medical staff: perhaps (he assumed) this was invented by the Jewish physicians themselves, in order to preserve some tiny shred of their professional dignity. Actually the Jewish prisoner-doctors were slave workers as well, employed in hard labor outside the camps, although allowed to carry a first-aid kit, and permitted to interrupt their work when a fellow-worker was injured, in order to dress his wounds.

In his task as a physician, Dr. Dvorjetski was forced to witness many of the horrid distortions of medicine during the Holocaust. The following are but a few examples. Ill prisoners in Klooga, one of the most infamous of camps, were forced out of the "Revier"[1] to work, even a short time after having undergone abdominal surgery. Prisoners with fever were not relieved of their work if their temperature was less than 39°C. The Jewish prisoner-physician Dr. Epstein, who requested bandages for Jews injured during work, was struck on his head for his "impudence." A German orderly murdered with a lethal injection a Jewish girl of four or five discovered by chance in the *Revier*.

The labor camps in Estonia were rife with epidemics, the most prevalent of which was spotted typhus, especially in winter because of the severe undernourishment and the freezing cold. The increase in lice heralded the appearance of the epidemic. Dr. Dvorjetski himself contracted the disease while at the camp in Korma. Among the symptoms of spotted typhus was the clouding of the patient's consciousness to the point of delirium, with fevered patients sometimes bursting into song and leaping from their sleeping bunks. Another symptom was gangrene of the legs. Such patients could not stand up and suffered from severe weakness which often preceded their death – whether by disease or by turning into apathetic and helpless "Muselmanns" – and were executed by the Germans. Sometimes patients suddenly got well, without any treatment. Those who were still capable of moving their limbs made every effort to go out and work, even when their temperature soared to 40°C. They knew that the Nazi doctors would hunt for prey, and that hospitalization in the camp *Revier* would probably hasten their being sent to their death in the next selection.

---

1   This was the usual nickname of the barracks where sick people were accommodated and supposed to be cared for medically. Very little was done for them in reality. *"Reviers"* existed in Auschwitz and other annihilation camps too.

The Jewish prisoner-doctors often helped patients to hide their illness, reporting them as suffering from influenza. In cases where such patients were ordered to have blood tests, the Jewish physicians stood the risk of having their subterfuge revealed. This was part of the continual contest of wits going on between them and the murderous Nazi doctors.

Also prevalent was dysentery. This diagnosis often served as a catchall term for all sorts of diarrhea. At times patients would suffer up to 30-40 daily bowel movements, often with bloody stools, and would die from exhaustion.

Other common diseases in the camps were pneumonia, skin rashes, brain concussions caused by work accidents, broken limbs (sometimes a result of the overseers' brutality), and frozen fingers or toes in the arduous winter work with insufficient footwear and no gloves.

The sick and injured were sent for treatment in the *Revier* of every camp. The conditions there were superficially tolerable: each one was staffed by prisoner-doctors and prisoner-nurses, the patients lying in reasonable comfort, and each *Revier* was provided with a small pharmacy and some supplies. From time to time, the Nazi head physician of all camps would arrive to make what was termed "a sanitary inspection." It quickly became evident that such arrangements were bogus. They were a trap for those weak in body or spirit; frequent selections were made among them. Most patients were "disposed" of. Again, the SS doctor was a murderer in a white smock, who used the cover of medical aid in order to make it easier for him to single out for annihilation the helpless patients.

The prisoner-doctor tried to outwit his Nazi inspector by doing exactly the opposite from the SS doctor and his orderlies: to preserve life as much as possible by hiding from them the cases of infectious diseases, by forging findings on illnesses, so as to disguise them in every way possible, by warning patients from being hospitalized in the *Reviers* and by encouraging them to go out to work in almost every situation – lest they fall into the hands of the SS doctors.

Among the techniques developed by Dr. Dvorjetski and others was the use of an ointment called Sapso that served as a substitute for iodine. The lesions typical in spotted typhus were masked in purple, and thus the telltale symptoms of the disease could be hidden for a time. The prisoner-doctors would also falsify medical records, such as fever charts. Before the visits of the Nazi doctors, they would even administer antipyretics to patients suffering from fever.

The spread of spotted typhus was fierce; it extended to a large proportion of the prisoners. The Germans, who greatly feared this epidemic, did not want to lose such large numbers of workers, and were finally forced to establish a special hospital, at Vaivara, where most of the typhus patients could be concentrated. Dr. Lazar Finkelstein, mentioned previously, headed the hospital. Thanks to his efforts, many patients recovered and returned to work reasonably quickly. Some were forced however to return on foot to the camp of their origin, and were not able to survive the rigors along the way. Dr. Finkelstein himself eventually perished.

Before the liquidation of the camps in Estonia with the advance of the Red Army in the beginning of 1944, selections were made for transfer of the prisoners to more distant camps. Dr. von Bothmann himself took pains to arrive at the Ereda camp, ordering the removal of almost a hundred prisoners in a rundown condition, to have them shot and have their corpses burned in a nearby wood. In another camp, Kivili, another large selection was made, eliminating hundreds of weakened prisoners. The SS men told them that they were being taken to a place of improved conditions, but instead, they were transferred by open train wagons to Vilnius, those who managed to survive this journey were driven to Ponary and killed there. Even prisoner-doctors, Dr. Leo Wikowiski among them, were exterminated in this action.

At the end of his personal journey of hardship, Dr. Dvorjetski was transferred to Dautmergen, a small camp in south Germany where, together with Polish prisoners captured after the failure of the Warsaw uprising, he worked quarrying raw materials for the manufacture of synthetic fuel – a job in which he had experience.

Another Jewish physician, the Czech Dr. Ernst Glaser, was interned in an adjacent slave labor camp in Mühldorf, and was able to save many of the Jewish workers whose health had deteriorated as a result of the long hours of strenuous work underground and insufficient nourishment. Dr. Glaser was allowed to receive leftover bones from the German staff kitchen as a personal gift, after successfully treating the medical problems of the deputy SS camp commandant. Instead of using the bones to cook soup for himself, Dr. Glaser charred them in an improvized oven, and ground them with bone marrow. The powder obtained was similar

in composition to the remedy known as *Carbo Animalis*, and served
to strengthen the health of many of the prisoners. This was a further
example of the resourcefulness and power of improvization shown by
Jewish prisoner-doctors in the camps.

When the Third Reich began to crumble in March and April of 1945,
many prisoners, including Dr. Dvorjetski, were driven on a hard march
to the Tyrol Mountains, possibly in order to build a fortified shelter for
Hitler. Together with 82 prisoners, Dr. Dvorjetski was able to exploit the
slackening of the guards (many of the German soldiers despaired of the
situation and deserted), and escaped to a forest near Saulgau, hiding for
several days until the Allied forces liberated them.

Upon coming to Israel after the war, Dr. Dvorjetski saw as his duty
the recording, preservation and research of Jewish medical heritage
in the ghettos and camps, and the documentation of the atrocities of
Nazi medicine. With the establishment of Bar-Ilan University in Israel,
Dr. Dvorjetski was appointed the first (and for many years, the only)
lecturer on this subject. In 1953 he was among the first recipients of the
State of Israel Prize, a reward for his unique contribution to historical
research. Dr. Marc Dvorjetski passed away in 1975.

Further reading

Yitzhak Arad. **Ghetto in Flames; the Struggle and Destruction of the Jews in Vilna.** New York: Holocaust Library, 1982.
Marc Dvorjetski. **Europe without Children; The Nazis' plans for Biological Destruction** (Hebrew). Jerusalem: Yad Vashem, 1958.
Marc Dvorjetski. **La Victoire du ghetto.** Paris: Editions France-Empire, 1962.

Chapter 11

Auschwitz

The very name Auschwitz Concentration Camp has become a veritable byword for the Jewish Holocaust. However, during its first year, from June 1940, few of the inmates were Jews. Initially, the internees were mainly Polish political prisoners, mostly of the intelligentsia, and included many physicians.

Auschwitz camp included medical installations from the beginning. Block 16 was designated as the internment place for ill prisoners. Here, Polish physicians were able to provide professional services to their compatriots. Blocks 14 and 15 were used as a quarantine for incoming prisoners. Towards the end of 1940, these three blocks were consolidated into what was known as "The Camp Clinic." It was primitive in its resources and medical equipment, and meager in its supply of medications. By contrast, the SS guards were provided with a small but well-equipped clinic at the edge of the camp, near their barracks.

On the first of March 1941, the SS supreme commander Heinrich Himmler visited the camp, then housing 10,000 inmates. He was impressed, particularly with its proximity to railroad junctions, and ordered its enlargement. He even approved the later plans of setting up an enormous camp in nearby Birkenau, with a capacity for 100,000 prisoners. At that time, it was not meant for Jews, but for Russian prisoners of war, with the Nazi preparations to attack the Soviet Union in progress. One of the possibilities taken into account was the availability of a large number of slave prisoners to be utilized as workers in the gigantic I. G. Farben industrial plant erected in Monowitz, not far from Auschwitz. Other German industrialists also eyed the seemingly unlimited supply of cheap forced labor. These considerations led to the founding of the whole Auschwitz complex of camps, housing over the years up to 150,000 prisoners.

The spring and summer months of 1941 were a time of great expansion of the Auschwitz camps in the spirit of Himmler's instructions. However, prisoner numbers far outgrew the building boom. The newly-built blocks were designed to hold four hundred, but in actuality had to accommodate many more; sometimes over a thousand prisoners crammed into them. The crowding was severely increased in the winter and spring of 1942, with the first mass deportations of Jews from Western Europe, following the decision on the "Final Solution of the Jewish Question."

Although the new gigantic camp at Birkenau had originally been planned as a Soviet prisoner-of-war camp, at that time, when it was in the process of completion, its new purpose gradually became clear: it was to serve as the largest extermination center for the Jewish people,[1] who had been sentenced to extinction. The Nazis even discovered a gas suitable for that design: Zyklon B, which, ironically, had been invented by the Jewish Nobel prize winner, the chemist Fritz Haber, as a pesticide. The mass killing with Zyklon B began in Birkenau in the spring of 1942,[2] initial experiments with this gas having already been carried out (on Soviet POWs) at the beginning of September 1941 within the old Auschwitz camp.

The involvement of SS physicians in the planned process of extermination was pivotal and the ultimate expression of the "medicalization" of the Holocaust. Only physicians were allowed to make the initial "selection" upon the arrival of the trains at the gates to the camp, making the choice between those to be sent immediately to be gassed and the more able-bodied to be kept alive for a certain period to be used as slave laborers. It was also the duty of Nazi physicians to oversee the extermination of the victims in the gas chambers. This was in accordance with the high standing of SS physicians in the Nazi bio-racial scheme. They were the ones responsible for carrying out the ethnic cleansing on an "industrial" scale in occupied Europe, as the heirs and followers of the special task forces (*Einsatzgruppen*) in occupied Soviet Union. In Auschwitz, SS physicians were also responsible for

---

1   According to the latest estimates (by the Polish historian Franciszek Piper) the number of Jews killed in Auschwitz-Birkenau reached one million souls. See his article in: **Anatomy of the Auschwitz death camp** (details at the end of this chapter).

2   One of the earliest documented murders by gas occurred in the middle of April 1942 and was described in detail at the Auschwitz trial in Germany, 1965. **Der Auschwitz Prozeß** (see at the end of this chapter), Vol. 1, pp. 459-463.

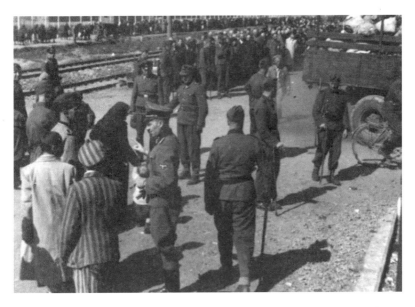

A "selection" on the Auschwitz railroad ramp. Courtesy of Yad Vashem Archives.

undertaking the ongoing selections of the forced laborers among those who had survived the initial selection at the entrance to the camp. The doctors signed their death certificates (mostly of fictitious causes) following the inevitable deterioration in their health after a few weeks or months of hard labor and poor conditions. All those responsibilities were in addition to their routine roles of epidemic prevention, medical care of camp personnel, including (at least theoretically) the Jewish slave laborers.

Six doctors held the position of Chief Physician of the Auschwitz complex of camps during its operation. Dr. Josef Mengele was not one of them (as is commonly believed). Mengele arrived at Auschwitz relatively late, towards the end of May 1943, directly from the Russian front, after having distinguished himself in battle, was wounded in combat, and awarded decorations. His military record on the Eastern Front added to his charisma. (Mengele will be dealt with in the next chapter.)

The most important and longest-serving of the six Chief Physicians at Auschwitz was Dr. Eduard Wirths. He took his duties seriously, trying to improve the health and hygiene conditions in Auschwitz. His

attitude towards Jewish physicians was relatively reasonable. Wirths'
appointment as Chief Physician in September 1942 led to an improvement
in the conditions of Jewish physicians (though developments of the war
at this time, particularly the German defeat at Stalingrad, also played
a role).

During the first period – with the beginning of the mass extermination
of the Jews – the fate of Jewish physicians arriving at Auschwitz was the
same as that of all Jews. All the Jewish inmates were to be murdered
sooner or later, making the subject of medical services for them seem
superfluous. Even those Jews who survived the initial selection at the
gates of the camp and were given a short reprieve from death as slave
laborers were not deemed worthy of real medical care. This was in
contrast to the Polish prisoners, who were allowed to maintain medical
services for themselves. For this reason, the Auschwitz authorities did
not bother to sift out or even register Jewish physicians arriving in
the transports. Hundreds of Jewish physicians were killed in the gas
chambers, their number representing the high proportion of Jews in the
medical profession in most European countries.

Appointment of Jewish physicians as "prisoner-doctors"

Towards the end of 1942 – around the time of the Nazi defeat in Stalingrad –
a significant change in the status of Jewish prisoner-physicians became
evident. The German command and leadership were haunted by the sudden
realization that victory was not assured. Consequently, they understood
they needed the skills of some of the Jews imprisoned in Auschwitz and
elsewhere, including the physicians. A reversal of practices concerning
able Jewish prisoners occurred. It became important to more efficiently
use the available slave labor than before, especially in the big industrial
plants manufacturing war materiel, set up in the new Auschwitz complex,
chiefly in Birkenau and Monowitz.

The hard work, the meager diet and the deplorable sanitation had
caused an enormous death rate and a continuous and swift turnover of
workers, most of them Jews, but also of Polish and Russian prisoners. At
first, the average life expectancy of slave workers did not exceed two or
three months, even though they had arrived physically robust enough to

survive the initial selection process. The camp administration grew aware of the need to ameliorate the conditions of these workers in order to lower their mortality rate. A marked improvement in food rations was out of the question (although there had been a slight increase in 1943-44), because of both the difficulties of supply and the opposition in principle of people like Hans Frank, the governor of Poland, who insisted on the necessity to get rid of all Jews – the sooner the better. The almost complete lack of fats and proteins in the official daily food rations (which never exceeded 1,400 calories) sapped the energies of all slave laborers save for those few who had some connections with the Germans or who stole from others. The lack of essential nourishment caused health problems. All internees lost weight rapidly; the prisoners' reserves of body fat and muscle tissue rapidly diminished. Many prisoners contracted dysentery due to the poor, and often contaminated, food and water. Most suffered from oedema and from skin ulcers and open wounds, especially in the lower limbs and the feet (because of ill-fitting footwear). The total absence of vitamins also took its toll. The lack of vitamins B and C aggravated the other symptoms among the weakening prisoners.

Obviously, the way to reduce mortality was to improve the medical care and hygiene in the camps, including preventing the spread of infectious diseases. The latter was of particular importance to the Germans, who were concerned with reducing the danger of disease spreading to their own quarters.

Towards the end of December 1942, the following directive was circulated by the SS Administration and Economy department, signed by Richard Glueck: "The Chief Camp Doctors must act with all means at their disposal to significantly lower the mortality rate in their camps." In spite of the decisive tone of this order, the obstacles to its implementation were many. SS physicians, who took an active part in the extermination process, were neither capable of, nor willing, to offer real medical care to their Jewish prisoner-patients. Their numbers were small, and the Nazi indoctrination they had received made them reluctant to provide medical help to Jews.

For these reasons, Dr. Wirths came to realize that Jewish prisoner-physicians should be allowed to treat their fellow Jewish prisoners. He granted them the title of "prisoner-physician" (*Häftlings-Arzt*). Previously, the Jewish doctors were referred to only as "caretaker"

(*Pfleger*) and were expected to work as hard as any other prisoner, although they carried first aid kits, and treated inmates injured during their slave labor.

Wirths recruited the help of Jewish physicians in controlling the spread of epidemics in Auschwitz. He had no scruples about employing for this purpose Jewish experts who were his prisoners, such as the famous serologist Prof. Ludwik Fleck.

Jewish doctors, as "prisoner-physicians," also provided medical care for the many Gypsy prisoners in Auschwitz. The success of the distinguished pediatrician Prof. Berthold Epstein and others in combating the Noma disease, which disfigured the faces of many Gypsy children, is well known.[3]

Some of the Jewish physicians worked within the new, larger and better-equipped hospital in Birkenau. A young and relatively inexperienced Jewish physician from Slovakia, Dr. Anna Weiss, was appointed head of its gynecological ward, provoking the animosity of the Polish physicians who had previously been in charge.

The mortality rate at the Birkenau hospital continued to be very high, due to poor diet and the too-brief periods of hospitalization and recuperation allowed the patients. Moreover, the imperative of most Nazi physicians, the wish to exterminate Jews, prevented the prolongation of the lives of Jewish patients, even after they had been treated successfully. Robert Lifton recounted in his book that complicated orthopedic operations, such as the setting of pelvic fractures, were carried out in the Birkenau hospital by Jewish experts, with SS physicians observing to learn the surgical procedures involved. These operations were successful – which did not however save the lives of their patients. They were sent afterwards to the gas chambers, camp authorities unwilling to wait for months for their complete recovery.

Most of the prisoner-doctors in Auschwitz were assigned to the horribly overcrowded barracks of the men and women slave workers, where a pitiful corner was allotted as a "*Revier,*" or sick room. Some blocks served wholly as *Reviers*, but the conditions there were no less dismal. The material resources available to physicians in the blocks were

---

3   Robert J. Lifton. **The Nazi Doctors** (Details at the end of this chapter), pp. 296-297.

extremely limited. They were not even provided with cloth bandages, and had to make do with poor substitutes, similar to toilet paper. On top of all this, the prisoner-physicians were themselves in a constant struggle for survival, under the supervision and at the mercy of the SS doctors overseeing them. This imposed further impediments to their attempts to provide medical aid to their Jewish patients.

The "prisoner-physicians'" dilemmas

While serving as prisoner-doctors, Jewish physicians wrestled with many difficult dilemmas, often at the very limits of medical ethics, and at times even contradicting them. For example, they were forced to decide who should be administered the paltry handful of medications provided to them at the start of each day: whether to give preference to the more seriously ill, or to those patients who had a chance for survival? Whether to report to the SS doctors that a patient needed an operation, when there was the real danger he would not be operated on, but instead sent to his death. Worst of all, they had to deal with the Nazi demands to prepare for them lists of fifty or a hundred patients, to be sent to the gas chambers in the next selection. The SS doctors tended to leave the prisoner-doctors with the never-ending process of choosing the next victims to be murdered. These were usually inmates whose strength had failed, or who had become physically exhausted and mentally apathetic, losing their hope and will to live, a state known as "Muselmann," or very ill people with little chance of regaining health.

The motives of the SS doctors in putting the burden of this horrible choice upon the Jewish physicians were clear: firstly they wished to rid themselves of the work required to sift through thousands of sick prisoners. Those SS doctors who sought to fulfill their duties with some claim of medical objectivity (and, according to Lifton's study,[4] a considerable number still considered themselves conscientious physicians), needed to devote many hours each day to the task. This required them to be in close proximity with the prisoners, and thus

---

4   Especially in part III of his book, **The Nazi Doctors,** with his concept of "The Auschwitz Self" helped by the mechanism of "doubling."

be vulnerable to infection. Naturally, the SS doctors were relieved to relegate this onerous task to Jewish prisoner-doctors, who were, besides, more familiar with the conditions of patients, with whom they spent day and night. The SS doctors sought to make the Jewish doctors their accomplices through shifting the onus of ethical responsibility onto as well, even if by coercion.

Taking part in the selections was doubtless the most excruciating duty of Jewish prisoner-physicians. It seems that nearly every one of them was forced to participate. Testimonies of survivors give the picture of their complex relations with the SS doctors. Even Nazi physicians understood that there was a limit to what they could demand of the prisoner-doctors, before meeting with a flat refusal.

Dr. Aharon Beilin testified during the Eichmann trial and spoke of his friend Dr. Globersohn, who had been assigned to serve as a physician for the *"Sonderkommando"* – the exclusive group of prisoners who assisted in the killings and the cremation of the bodies and cleaned the gas chambers. The Germans realized that members of the *Sonderkommando* were witnesses to the secrets of annihilation, secrets they needed to take to their graves. Correspondingly, they were generally liquidated after six months of service. The *Sonderkommando* enjoyed better rations, living conditions and medical care, in order to preserve their capacity for work. When the SS commander of the *Sonderkommando* units, *Hauptscharführer* Otto Moll, chanced upon Dr. Globersohn attending to the Gypsies in their section of the camp, he took him with the aim of making him the *Sonderkommando* prisoner-doctor. The Jewish physician refused. In an attempt to evade Moll's order, Dr. Globersohn swallowed sleeping pills in order to commit suicide – but the dose was apparently insufficient, and he survived only to be severely beaten by Moll as punishment. Dr. Beilin saw him two days later, badly bruised but steadfast in his refusal. Moll then went over to Birkenau, where the beaten physician had been taken, and brutally flogged him to death.

Under such coercion, most Jewish physicians acceded to assisting in the selections. One of the last surviving doctors interviewed by me, Dr. P. R., gave this simple justification: when she was forced to select the victims, they usually were people who had minimal hope for survival, from a medical viewpoint. On the other hand, when the Germans were left with the choice, there was a good chance that, out of capriciousness, laziness or ignorance, they would select inmates who were capable of survival. Such was the case with a tall, young, blonde woman whom she had helped terminate an unwanted pregnancy. Shortly afterwards, although her medical condition was satisfactory, that woman was selected by an SS doctor for the gas chambers, on the curious pretext that a Jewish woman who was so Aryan-looking should not continue to live – since this so obviously contradicted the Nazi racial doctrine...

Some Jewish physicians reached a certain unspoken agreement with the SS doctors: they would not point out the hopeless cases, but would indicate the larger group of those still capable of surviving. The SS doctor would then reach his own conclusions, and send the members of the other group to their deaths.

Jewish physicians saving prisoners

Often the lives of prisoners in Auschwitz were saved by Jewish doctors, through their medical care, their moral support and their efforts to foil the SS doctors. Doctors would eliminate or fake medical findings which could place the patient's life in jeopardy. According to surviving testimonies, laboratory findings, which would otherwise have doomed the patient, were often hidden or forged. Severe diagnoses or pathological findings were "lost" or altered.

There were times when Jewish physicians even made attempts to hide outbreaks of contagious disease among patients. In such cases, they confronted an even more complicated dilemma: on the one hand, they knew that involving the SS doctor in this meant an almost automatic death sentence for the infected patient. On the other hand, if they let the patient go unreported they endangered the entire barrack, the healthy and the ill. Usually the Jewish doctors were stringent and took into consideration the common good.

Sometimes, mere words of encouragement and moral support from a Jewish doctor made all the difference. Such was the case of the Polish-born physician, Dr. Lowitsch (who had studied medicine in France). He stopped his colleague, who had lost his whole family upon arrival from Thessaloniki, from committing suicide by running towards the electric fence. He convinced him by saying: "Do not allow these German scoundrels to be happy by killing everyone of us. Let us stand firm and outlive those criminals."[5] True to his word, both doctors survived.

Quite a few pregnant women arrived at Auschwitz. It was common for those in their first months to pass the initial selection undetected. If the evidence of the pregnancy became unmistakable, however, the lives of both the mother and the fetus were doomed. Several Jewish women physicians tried to save the mothers' lives by performing abortions in secret.

The gynecologist, Dr. Gisela Perl, organized this undercover activity. She was born in a traditional Jewish home in Sziget, Hungary, and gained experience in abortions and obstetrics in a small hospital within the local ghetto. In May 1944, she was transferred to Auschwitz with her parents and dentist husband, all of whom (dentistry not being needed in Auschwitz) were consigned to the gas chambers. She was ordered to manage a tiny hospital – in effect, a *Revier* – set up in Block 15 of Birkenau. Dr. Perl and her fellow-workers – four physicians and four nurses – had no medical supplies or instruments. One corner of the *Revier* was isolated as an operating area, separated from the rest by several boards. Apart from a wooden table, a few pairs of rusty scissors, and one knife which had to be resharpened on a simple stone after each use, no other implement was available to this small medical team.

Dr. Perl made use of the *Revier* to hide pregnant women, disguising them as pneumonia cases. Such women were transferred to her from all over the camp with the aid of a network of Jewish women doctors, sending them to the *Revier* to undergo abortions and curettage in the dead of night.

As a religious woman, Dr. Perl knew that Jewish Law permitted the sacrificing of a fetus when the mother's life was endangered. She was thus particularly anxious that her patients who had undergone abortions and premature childbirths should survive. As she wrote in her memoirs,[6] "Every time when kneeling down in the mud, dirt [...] to perform a delivery without instruments, without water, without the most elementary requirements of hygiene, I prayed to God to help me save the mother or

5   According to the testimony of Tzvi Michaeli, **Yad Vashem,** VT-1739.
6   **I was a Doctor in Auschwitz,** New York: International Universities Press, 1948 (reprint: 1987) p. 81.

I would never touch a pregnant woman again. […] God was good to me. By a miracle, which to every doctor must sound like a fairy tale, every one of these women recovered and was able to work, which, at least for a while, saved her life."

Further reading

Israel Gutman and Michael Berenbaum (eds.). **Anatomy of the Auschwitz Death Camp**. Bloomington and Indianapolis, Ind.: Indiana University Press, 1994.

Ernst Klee. **Auschwitz, die NS-Medizin und ihre opfer**. Frankfurt am Main: S. Fischer, 1997.

Hermann Langbein. **Der Auschwitz Prozeß; Eine Dokumentation.** 2 Vols. Wien: Europa Verlag, 1965.

Robert Jay Lifton, **The Nazi doctors; Medical Killing and the Psychology of Genocide**. New York: Basic Books, 1986 [German edition: 1988].

Chapter 12

Medical Experiments

In the German city of Lübeck, in 1930, a dreadful incident occurred. An experimental BCG vaccine against tuberculosis, without proper pre-testing, was administered to a number of babies and small children. As a result, over seventy infants died within a month. The Jewish physician, Dr. Julius Moses, mentioned earlier as the one warning almost prophetically against the distortion of medical values by the Nazis, was also a voice in the wilderness against the experiments carried out in Lübeck.[1]

Following that incident, Dr. Moses drafted a list of principles for the testing of new preparations, and for medical experiments generally. These emphasized the importance of a complete explanation to the candidates or, in the case of children, their guardians, and the obtaining of their agreement – nowadays known as "informed consent." Dr. Moses suggested these new regulations to German parliamentary bodies, but they never became law. The Nazis came to power, and Moses' labor was in vain. Only in the Nuremberg Code, adopted in 1947 following the Nazi Doctors' Trials, were these suggestions from Dr. Moses and others incorporated.

The Nazi physicians used people they considered of "inferior value" for unscrupulous experimentation. Within the T4 Institute in Brandenburg, quasi-experimental use was made of the brains of "euthanized" retarded patients. Worse still, the prisoners of the concentration and extermination camps were subjected to shocking experimentation while still alive.

---

1   Daniel S. Nadav. "**'Death Dance of Lübeck': Julius Moses and the German Guidelines for Human Experimentation, 1930,**" in: Volker Roelcke and Giovanni Maio (eds.). **Twentieth Century Ethics of Human Subjects Research.** Stuttgart: Franz Steiner, 2004.

Medical experiments in concentration camps

The medical experiments carried out in concentration camps have been reliably documented. They involved about 8,000 people – though there is little doubt that the real number of victims was much greater. Nearly every one of those human subjects in many experiments perished, preventing us from receiving first-hand accounts.

Some experiments, ignoring their brutality, had a certain level of objective justification. In Dachau, Luftwaffe doctors examined the effects of high-altitude air pressure on the health of POWs, mostly Russians but also Jews. They were subjected to simulations of high altitudes within pressure chambers, without any protection. It was possible for the researchers to learn at what altitude pilots needed to wear oxygen masks from the signs of distress (and even death) of the subjects. These experiments were filmed and the footage was used as evidence at the Nuremberg Trials. In other experiments, people were immersed alive in icy water, different means were attempted to revive them, and prisoners were forced to drink salt water. The goal of such experiments was to find out how German airmen could best survive when downed over the North Atlantic in freezing and salty water.

Experiments, often on Jews, were carried out in Auschwitz and other camps. Such experiments had perhaps a slight, albeit questionable justification – but the methods used violated even the most tenuous ethical norms. Prisoners were deliberately infected with various diseases, such as typhus and infectious hepatitis, and afterwards were subjected to assorted, and sometimes bizarre, treatments. An extensive series of experiments with typhus was carried out in Buchenwald, at the initiative of the SS chiefs of medicine, Prof. Joachim Mrugowsky and Dr. Karl Genzken. One group of victims was inoculated with a variety of agents in universal use; a second group remained untreated so as to be kept as a control group. A third group was infected with the disease right at the start of the experiment, so that live bacteria could be extracted from their bodies in order to subsequently infect others. These experiments involved 729 subjects, of whom at least 154 perished.

Similarly ruthless experiments were carried out in other concentration camps; victims were purposefully injured with chemical agents such as phosphorus, or even gas warfare agents such as mustard gas

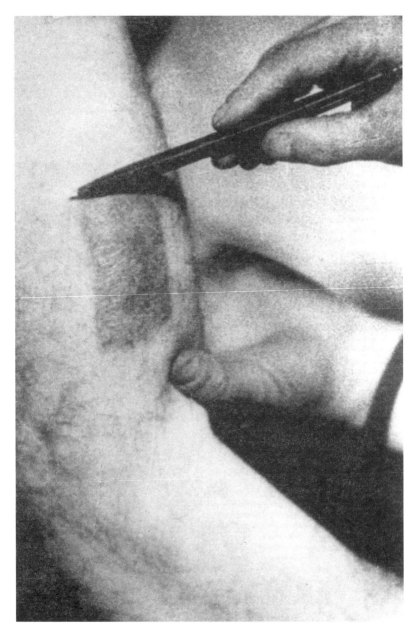

A phosphorus burn inflicted on a prisoner. Courtesy of Yad Vashem Archives.

or phosgene, and the effectiveness of various treatments was tested. The man responsible for promoting these experiments was Hitler's personal physician, Dr. Karl Brandt, who had been involved before in the "euthanasia" program. In June 1942 he was appointed Reich Commissioner for Health and Sanitation in Germany, with responsibility for the armed services and all SS research institutes.

Israeli scholar Dr. Nava Cohen recounts an unusual experiment conducted in the women's concentration camp at Ravensbrück.[2] The victims were 75 Polish political prisoners. The doctor responsible for this was Dr. Karl Gebhardt, the chief SS surgeon and Himmler's personal physician. It was he who unsuccessfully treated Reinhard Heydrich for a week, after the assassination attempt by the Czech underground in May 1942. Some doctors claimed that he should have used sulfanilamide, a new medicine at the time, which would have prevented the infection and gangrene which led to Heydrich's death. Himmler demanded that Gebhardt should test this out himself. Gebhardt had, understandably, a personal interest in proving his detractors wrong. So he made a deliberate effort to inflict especially severe infections on the victims of this experiment. Many of them died or were maimed for life as a consequence.

Also in Ravensbrück, the leg bones of healthy young women were deliberately fractured in order to test on them various curative procedures. During these experiments, even entire bones and other tissues were extracted, in an attempt to implant them in wounded SS men lying in a nearby hospital.

Other experiments performed in Nazi concentration camps were meant to strengthen the evidence for the Nazi ideological distinctions between Aryans and assumed inferior races, or to assist in sterilizing and exterminating Jews and other unwanted elements.

Additional experiments were meant to aid the fostering of the Aryan race. This, for instance, was one of the chief motives of Dr. Mengele, who studied with assiduous fascination the phenomenon of multiple births. He was hoping to find the genetic cause for the birth of twins and

2   Nava Cohen. **"Medical Experiments,"** in **Encyclopedia of the Holocaust,** pp. 957-966. New York: Macmillan, 1990.

thereby enable the Germans to recover more quickly the demographic losses of the war.

Dr. Mengele's experiments

Dr. Mengele, who became known as the "Auschwitz Angel of Death" and who was the very emblem of the distorted medical Nazi practices, was born in 1911 and there is no doubt he was a talented man. He achieved at

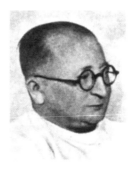

Prof. Carl Clauberg. Courtesy of Yad Vashem Archives.

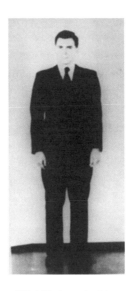

Dr. Josef Mengele. Courtesy of Yad Vashem Archives.

a very young age two doctorates: in philosophy and medicine. Aspiring
to an academic career, he became an outstanding assistant to one of the
devotees of the theories of heredity: Prof. Otmar von Verschuer, director
of the Kaiser Wilhelm Institute of Anthropology, Human Heredity and
Eugenics in Frankfurt.

Mengele joined the Nazi Party and the SS in the thirties. From June
1940 he served with distinction as a physician in the SS field units and
was wounded in battle. At the end of May 1943 he was transferred to
Auschwitz, where he gained much appreciation from his fellow SS
colleagues because of his military past and his charismatic personality.
A short time afterwards, he was appointed the Camp Doctor (*Lagerarzt*)
of Birkenau. At the same time, he directed the experiments in Block 10
in the Auschwitz main camp. Mengele was technically the subordinate
of the Auschwitz chief physician, Dr. Eduard Wirths, but was generally
considered by many to be the more powerful of the two. Camp survivors
remember Mengele as the man who single-handedly conducted the
"selections" at the gates of Auschwitz. But he certainly had helpers. It
would not have been possible even for Mengele to have been physically
present on the ramp at the camp gates for 24 hours a day.

Other Nazi physicians who took part in the selections respected
Mengele's order that he receive all twins arriving from each transport.
According to reliable estimates, his researches involved at least 1,500
pairs of twins.[3] A small number of them survived when Auschwitz was
liberated by the Russian Army in January 1945. Mengele showed interest
in other peculiar cases: dwarfs, or others of abnormal shapes, seeking in
them characteristics typical of the "genetically inferior" Jewish race.

Mengele continued his ties with von Verschuer and the Kaiser
Wilhelm Institutes, sending them, from time to time, samples of his
Auschwitz "findings"; decapitated heads and other tissue samples taken
from bodies of "inferior" victims. On his initiative, the eyes of Gypsy
victims were injected with materials designed to make the color of their
naturally brown eyes lighter and blue. Then they were gouged out. He
took care to send to the collection of Prof. August Hirt in Strassburg a

3   Some of them were not actual twins, rather brothers or sisters who looked similar
and were represented by their mothers as twins in order to save them from
annihilation.

126 Chapter 12

whole array of Jewish skeletons, and so leave anthropological evidence of their inherent so-called human inferiority.

The part of "prisoner doctors" in experiments

Mengele's interest in various medical experiments led to his being delegated responsibility for Block 10 in the old Auschwitz camp, where these experiments were carried out. Among other things, these experiments included irradiation of Jewish men and women's genitalia, in order to sterilize them. Prof. Carl Clauberg and Dr. Horst Schumann were behind these experiments, but Mengele assisted them greatly. Himmler, in the background, was interested in these experiments as well and ensured the researchers had all means and manpower available to them. He hoped that these experiments in human sterilization would allow the Germans to exploit the slave labor potential of the Slavic races and still prevent them from reproducing.

Mengele made use of the expertise of the Jewish pathologist Miklos Nyiszli, who performed autopsies on the victims of Clauberg and Schumann, as well as on those of Mengele himself, including the twins. Dr. Nyiszli, who survived Auschwitz, wrote an important account of his work in Block 10 which included testimony of the complex and sadistic personality of Mengele himself. He details how Mengele would pamper the children among "his" twins, lay a chocolate on their bed in the evening – and coldheartedly order their murder the next day, so that he could compare the inner organs of each with that of his sibling who had been dispatched beforehand.

One of the Jewish physicians who were taken to work in Block 10 was the surgeon and gynecologist, Dr. Maximilian Samuel. Robert Lifton, in his research, has lambasted Dr. Samuel as a "Jewish medical collaborator [...] the one Jewish doctor I know of."[4] Closer examination reveals the injustice of this statement. Dr. Samuel was eventually put to death by the Germans for sabotaging their experiments, though it is possible that, for a while, he did show loyalty to his German masters. At any rate, the story of his life is a demonstration of the terrible dilemmas

4   **The Nazi Doctors**, p. 250.

facing Jewish physicians during the Holocaust and, in particular, those of the "prisoner-doctors" in the death camps.

Dr. Samuel was born in 1880 in a suburb of Cologne, maintaining there a gynecological and surgical clinic for thirty years, until 1938. In World War I he served as a military doctor and was awarded decorations for bravery. On returning to Cologne after the war, he took part as a confirmed German patriot in resistance to the French occupation in the Rhineland in the early twenties. Samuel, a tall and sturdy man, was a sports enthusiast, specializing also in sports medicine. He was highly respected as a practitioner and as a generous person. According to the evidence collected in Cologne, thanks to the efforts of Benno Müller-Hill, he treated many women free of charge, at times even slipping them parcels of food.

With the advent of Nazism, Samuel's life became full of hardship. In spite of this, he did not hasten to leave Germany, as did other Jewish physicians. In July 1938, as with all Jewish physicians, his license to practice medicine was revoked, and he was forced to close his clinic. When the Gestapo came to arrest him on November 1938, during *Kristallnacht*, he showed his resourcefulness by quickly donning his military uniform replete with war decorations and confronted the situation with aplomb. The Gestapo agents were embarassed and left to receive instructions. That same night, Samuel fled with his family to nearby Belgium, passing from there to France, where he lived for a few years. In August 1942 he was caught, however, and finally sent to Auschwitz, with his wife and only daughter.

In Auschwitz, his wife was immediately sent to the gas chambers. Sixty-two year old Dr. Samuel, along with his daughter of eighteen, Lieselotte, were among the few who survived the selection. Being a physician apparently saved him, for that was the time that the Nazis had begun utilizing Jewish "prisoner-doctors."

Samuel and his daughter were taken to Monowitz to work in the Buna plant for the production of artificial rubber, still in construction at the time. Samuel was allowed to work at the factory's clinic. The factory owners were concerned with preserving the work capabilities of their forced laborers, and therefore provided a clinic much better supplied than other places in Auschwitz. Among his many deeds here, Samuel managed to save the life of a Czech political prisoner, Rudolf Ruebke, by administering him injections of Salvarsan.

The relative freedom of movement in the camp Samuel enjoyed, and the bigger food rations he received, enabled him to help his daughter hold out in the heavy forced labor demanded of her. From time to time, he managed to see her, to encourage her and bring her some food.

To Samuel's misfortune, Mengele happened to hear of him. His expertise as gynecologist and surgeon was needed in Block 10, where experiments in sterilizing Jewish women were carried out. Jewish women transported from the Greek port city of Thessaloniki were arriving, and Dr. Horst Schumann had promised Himmler that he would be able to sterilize a thousand Jewesses a day with an X-ray procedure he was trying out. This way, the barren women could be used as a work-force, without the worry of their conceiving. The procedure, however, still needed to be verified.

In the spring of 1943, Samuel was forced to become part of the team. His task, together with the Polish physician, Wladislaw Dering, was to remove for examination parts of the reproductive organs of women who had undergone severe X-ray irradiation. Large parts of the uterus, with one (and sometimes both) of the ovaries, were excised and sent for examination, to observe the effectiveness of the irradiations. The X-ray procedure proved to be inadequate to ensure the complete sterilization of the victims. The operations, however, greatly endangered the women's fertility, and sometimes even their lives. Many women came down with infections because of the operations or irradiations, and died after terrible suffering.

Dr. Wirths also made use of Dr. Samuel's services. Together with his brother Helmut, he conducted dubious investigations into cervical cancer. They had Samuel remove parts of cervices from women who had been treated with various materials against the spread of cancer, after the cervix had been photographed with the aid of a colposcope. The removed tissue samples were sent to Helmut Wirths' laboratory in Hamburg.

As is evident, Samuel served both Wirths and Mengele in parallel, and for a time discharged his duties to the satisfaction of both. This may be explained by his concern for his daughter, who was suffering serious malnutrition in Monowitz. In his despair, he even wrote a letter to Himmler, in which he summarized his service to Germany in the war and afterwards and begged to have his daughter's life spared. It is almost certain, however, that the letter never reached its addressee. Samuel remained helpless in the face of his daughter's plight, until she died in autumn 1943. Apparently he then decided he had nothing more to lose, and sabotaged the experiments performed on the Thessaloniki Jewesses, helping them, to the best of his abilities, to avoid their dire results.

From the testimonies of three women kept in Yad Vashem (Jerusalem), it appears that Samuel disguised his subterfuge by performing sham procedures. He didn't extract the womb or ovaries. Instead, he made harmless incisions and removed innocuous parts, which did not impair the women's fertility. According to Rebecca Aharon's testimony,[5] for example, Samuel "performed many operations on four women, and did nothing wrong, only opened their bellies, so that it would appear that he had operated on them, but didn't do them harm. All of them have children." One of the women mentioned by Aharon was Aliza Baruch, who married after the war, and had a boy and a girl in Israel. Rebecca Aharon herself was not operated upon by Dr. Samuel, but by someone else (probably Dr. Dering) and remained barren.

But at the end, in September or October 1943, SS doctors started suspecting that Samuel was evading their instructions, and on a return examination of one of the women, they realized that Samuel had been fooling them. He was taken on that very same day to Birkenau and was put to death.

From the tragic story of Dr. Samuel, it is possible to see the difficult conditions of many Jewish physicians, who were faced with impossible dilemmas. Was Samuel really a collaborator, as Lifton claimed? His heroic end places such a conclusion in doubt. Is it possible, however, for those of us who have never had to face such horror and such awful choices to pass judgement on physicians who found themselves in this predicament? Primo Levi, the writer and Holocaust survivor, wisely refused to blame anyone who had found himself in what he termed "the gray zone." In Auschwitz prisoners had to struggle for survival while wrestling with their consciences in conditions of unimaginable hardship. For those who have not experienced such excruciating impasses and have never been faced with such unimaginable wickedness, it is advisable to show humility. We should refrain from voicing criticism of the choices

---

5   **Yad Vashem**, 0.3/4564.

made in the face of that horror. Instead, we need to show understanding of, and empathy for, the nearly impossible position these imprisoned physicians found themselves in. They were also victims of hellish evil.

Further reading

Hermann Langbein. **People in Auschwitz.** Chapel Hill: University of North Carolina, 2004.

Alexander Mitscherlich and F. Mielke. **Doctors of Infamy; the Story of Nazi Medical Crimes.** New York: H. Schuman, 1949 [a translation of the German book which appeared in the same year].

Miklos Nyiszli. **Auschwitz: a Doctor's Eyewitness Account.** New York: Fredrick Fell, 1960.

R. Osnowski (ed.). **Menschenversuche, Wahnsinn und Wirklichkeit.** Köln: Volksblatt Verlag, 1988.

Chapter 13

Doctors' Trials at Nuremberg

After their victory in World War II, the Allies put on trial those of the Nazi leadership captured alive. Starting from October 1945, their trial was conducted before a specially created military court in Nuremberg.

During these trials, the idea was posited to initiate a separate trial against the Nazi physicians. The awfulness of their crimes – at least when pertaining to the medical experiments – was already common knowledge. Some of the more senior criminal physicians, principally Mengele, had managed to escape or commit suicide. Mengele found his final refuge in South America. In addition to the difficulties of locating all the Nazi doctors, the prosecutors did not get the cooperation of the other victorious powers, which had typified the Allies on the eve of the original Nuremberg trials. In the end, the Americans conducted the trial against the Nazi doctors alone. The court action is officially known hence as "United States of America vs. Karl Brandt *et al.*"

The Nuremberg Doctors' Trials were opened with the presentation of the allegations against the defendants on the 25th of October 1946 and continued until the 20th of August 1947. The trial generally provoked much less interest than the trials of the Nazi chiefs, which had occurred a year before and captured the attention of worldwide interest. Only twenty Nazi physicians, nearly all SS doctors, stood trial. Among them was Karl Brandt, Hitler's personal physician and Reich's Commissoner for Health and Sanitation. Viktor Brack was also put on trial. Though not a physician, as chief administrative officer in Hitler's chancellery he had responsibility for the "euthanasia" program and was deemed accountable. The directors and physicians of the institutes of the medical murder, in which "euthanasia" had been carried out, such as Imfried Eberl and Friedrich Mennecke, were absent from the dock. Their crimes were hard to prove at that time due to the unavailability of detailed information on what had taken place in their institutions. However, materials concerning the main

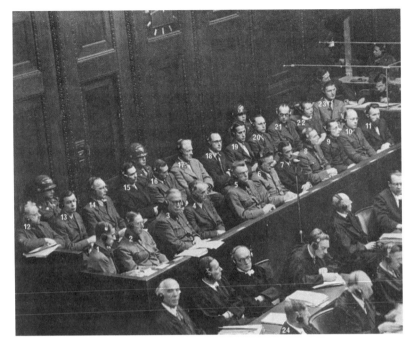

Nazi physicians on trial in Nuremberg (No.1 – Karl Brandt). Courtesy of Yad
Vashem Archives.

designs of the euthanasia program were in the hands of the prosecution.
In addition, some of the persons involved in medical experiments in the
concentration camps were indictable, since the documentation had already
been partially collected. The deeds were easy to prove, particularly when
survivors, such as men and women sterilized in Auschwitz, were still alive
and could testify to their injuries and their mental suffering. It was much
more difficult to clarify the entire medicalization process of the Holocaust,
which involved so many physicians. The truth about the Ghettoization
under the guise of medical justifications (like in Warsaw, for example),
and the employment of knowledge gained from the T4 program in
operating extermination camps was little known at the time, and pertinent
documents were only uncovered much later.

   Thus the impression was formed that only a few doctors – about
fifty or one hundred at most – were involved in medical crimes. Those
responsible for medical organizations that "purged" all Jewish physicians

in the 1930s, denying them their livelihood, were not brought to trial. The severity of such deeds were not considered as "crimes against humanity" – the main accusation (and a new category in the history of international law) against the defendants in the Nuremberg Trials.

In addition to those directly involved in "euthanasia" and medical experiments, some of those appointed to key medical positions in the SS were also put on trial, like Prof. Mrugowsky, chief of the Hygienic Institute of the Waffen SS, and some administrative heads, such as the aforementioned Brack.

The trial and the defendants' reactions

Even though some of the Germans involved in medical crimes had been arrested, almost from the start difficulties arose in the legal procedures against them, precisely because there was no judicial precedent to the severity of their deeds. It was impossible to classify them into one of the accepted categories of international law at the time. That law had not recognized such terrible acts on the part of physicians towards their defenseless victims. On the other hand, Nazi ideology provided justifications, distorted as they were, for the criminal actions of those physicians. They had a duty to obey orders (a claim used by Eichmann in his Jerusalem trial). Further, they argued the medical need to investigate ways of dealing with unsolved medical problems arising in part from military necessity – like phosphorus burns or the speedy warming of the human body after a person had fallen into freezing water.

The defendants' attorneys tried to make use of a variety of such arguments in favor of their clients. They even made accusations against the Americans themselves, who also conducted unpleasant experiments on jailed prisoners. One such research program sought a cure for hepatitis, the cause of suffering for many American soldiers during the war. Indeed, in the absence of an accepted and binding code for conducting human experiments, many countries availed themselves of the license – even in the democratic West – of carrying out experiments, which from our viewpoint today would be regarded as unacceptable. Prisoners were not given adequate information about the dangers to which they were to be exposed in the conduct of the experiment, and their consent was often obtained in return for some minimal improvement in the conditions of their imprisonment.

In his opening address Brigadier-General Telford Taylor, U.S. counsel for the prosecution in the Nazi Doctors' Trial, emphasized the need to condemn the Nazi physicians' deeds as "barbarous and criminal." He used the well-known statement of another American prosecutor (Robert H. Jackson) in the trial of the Nazi chiefs the previous year:

> The wrongs which we seek to condemn and punish have been so calculated, so malignant, and so devastating, that civilization cannot tolerate their being ignored, because it cannot survive their being repeated.

The details in the doctors' trials – evidence of medical experiments and "euthanasia" – were plentiful. A mountain of documents served as proof of the guilt of most of the defendants.

Despite the overwhelming evidence, the rights of the defendants to a fair legal defense were protected. First-rank German lawyers attempted to justify, or at least to offer explanations for their actions, in the light of exigency of the Nazi dictatorship. The defendants were also given the right to be heard.

In order to justify his deeds, Karl Brandt, an impressive-looking man, put forth claims and reasons of a semi-philosophical nature. He attempted to evade the expected death sentence with a mixture of sanctimoniousness and self-pity. His last words before the Court were:

> There is a word which seems so simple – order; and how colossal are its implications. How immeasurable are the conflicts which hide behind the word obey. Both affected me, obey and order, and both imply responsibility [...]. The prosecution has brought the charge of crime and murder and they have raised the question of my guilt. [...] friends and patients [could] shield me and speak well of me, saying I had helped and I had healed. There would be many examples of my actions during danger and my readiness to help. All that is now useless. As far as I am concerned I shall not evade these charges. But the attempt to vindicate myself as a man is my duty towards all who believe in me personally, who trusted

in me and who relied upon me as a man as well as a doctor and a superior.

Following this, Brandt made reference to the subject of medical experiments, claiming:

I have never regarded human experiments as a matter of course, not even when no danger was entailed. But I affirm the necessity for them on grounds of reason. I know that opposition will arise. I know things that disturb the conscience of a medical man, and I know the inner distress that afflicts one when ethics of every form are decided by an order or [military] obedience.

Brandt even tried to turn to his favor the words of Pastor Bodelschwing, who had taken retarded children from his hands at "Bethel" for extermination in the T4 program. Bodenschwing was quoted as claiming that Brandt was not a criminal, but an idealist! Brandt showed no repentance for his deeds. He testified that if he were asked again his view of "euthanasia," he would still approve of it. He alleged that the "euthanasia" had not been murder (undoubtedly a false claim), for "death can be a deliverance and liberation from a lingering suffering." Typical of the Nazis, Brandt cynically used phrases meant to justify "euthanasia," which was in reality the planned brutal mass murder of helpless victims carried out by the T4 operators. Brandt admitted that he "bears the responsibility with a heavy heart – but it is not a responsibility for a crime."

When Brandt's death sentence was announced, he tried to avoid his execution with an original offer: he was willing to endure experiments of a similar severity to that which his victims had undergone. This offer, and a similar one from Gerhard Rose, was rejected. Brandt and his co-condemned – seven in all – were hanged in Landsberg prison at the beginning of June, 1948. Some of the condemned tried to evade the execution and took their own lives in their prison cells.

In his trial, Karl Brandt totally ignored the Nazi doctrinal motivation for his acts. Several other Nazi physicians, however, admitted that their deeds were necessitated by their faith in essentially political goals.

Prof. Paul Rostock, a famous surgeon who was finally acquitted, admitted that he and others were not strong enough to deal with "a science directed by politics," especially when the real issues were so "artfully" distorted and manipulated – as he phrased it.

Dr. Kurt Blome, who served as deputy leader of the Reich physicians Association, admitted that he, like the rest of the German people, had become enthralled by what he called "Hitler's trap." He claimed that only during the trial did he begin to understand what a criminal regime he had served.

Some of the accused, such as senior SS physician Helmut Poppendick, tried to put the blame on others, who were not tried, particularly Dr. Ernst Grawitz, the SS chief physician, who committed suicide at the end of the war. Poppendick described the behavior of Grawitz as "inhuman." During the war, Grawitz had served as president of the German Red Cross – an organization that did nothing for the victims of the distorted medical practices; on the contrary, he initiated some of the cruelest experiments in the concentration camps. Grawitz did not even protest the fact that vehicles bearing the Red Cross were used in Auschwitz to transport the containers of the "Zyklon B" poison pellets to the gas chambers.

Viktor Brack, one of the originators of the idea of sterilizing Jews and forced laborers, tried to play the innocent with his ridiculous claim that he had raised the issue to save the lives of Jews. He was unable to bring proof or witnesses in support of his claim, and was condemned to death.

There were other physicians, like Siegfried Ruff and Georg Weltz, both responsible for medical research institutes of the German air force, who pointed to their decisive opposition to experiments conducted in Dachau, meant to test human endurance in low-pressure atmospheric conditions in high altitudes, and the ability to survive in freezing water. They proved during their trial that they had succeeded in convincing their superiors of the uselessness of these experiments, which had already cost the lives of many Jewish and Russian prisoners of war, and to have them stopped. Both physicians were acquitted.

The practical outcome of these trials of the Nazi doctors – over and above the meting out of justice – was the drawing up of the Nuremberg Code in 1947. This was the first series of internationally sanctioned regulations, governing the proper conduct of human medical experiments.

The Nuremberg Code and its implications

Through writing the Nuremberg Code, the lessons learned from the distorted and perverse inhumanity of the Nazi medical experiments were addressed. Never again should human beings be treated as subjects without proper attention paid to their rights. The document contains "ten commandments," as follows:

1. *The voluntary consent of the human subject is absolutely essential.* (The meaning here is unambiguous: each candidate for any experiment must receive an explanation beforehand of the nature of the experiment, of the dangers and difficulties involved, and must give his free agreement to his participation. It reminds us of Julius Moses' proposals back in 1930).
2. *The experiment should be such as to yield fruitful results for the good of society, unprocurable by other methods or means of study, and not random or unnecessary in nature.*
3. *The experiment should be so designed and based on the results of animal experimentation and a knowledge of the natural history of the disease or other problems under study that the anticipated result will justify the performance of the experiment.*
4. *The experiment should be so conducted as to avoid all unnecessary physical and mental suffering and injury.*
5. *No experiment should be so conducted where there is an a priori reason to believe that death or disabling injury will occur; except, perhaps, in those experiments where the experimental physicians also serve as subjects.*
6. *The degree of risk to be taken should never exceed that determined by the humanitarian importance of the problem to be solved by the experiment.*
7. *Proper preparations should be made and adequate facilities provided to protect the experimental subject against even remote possibilities of injury, disability, or death.*
8. *The experiment should be conducted only by scientifically qualified persons. The highest degree of skill and care should be required through all stages of the experiment of those who conduct or engage in the experiment.*

9. *During the course of the experiment, the human subject should be at liberty to bring the experiment to an end, if he has reached the physical or mental state where continuation of the experiment seems to him to be impossible.*

10. *During the course of the experiment, the scientist in charge must be prepared to terminate the experiment at any stage, if he has probable cause to believe, in the exercise of good faith, superior skill and careful judgment required of him that a continuation of the experiment is likely to result in injury, disability, or death to the experimental subject.*

The Nuremberg Code served as a declaration of human rights, and a suitable reply to their flagrant breach in the Nazi human experiments. The Code revealed several weaknesses, however. As it stood originally, the Nuremburg Code put obstacles in the path of legitimate medical research. The need to provide suitable information to every participant in any experiment, for example, served to prevent experiments involving (and therefore, for the benefit of) children or persons with certain mental limitations. As a result, the need arose to amend the Code in such a way as to enable the legal guardians of such persons to give their consent in their stead, when their charges are not competent to do so. Two decades later, in 1964, the World Medical Association issued the Declaration of Helsinki, dealing chiefly with human experimentation. This Declaration has been amended five times to date.

The influence of the Nuremberg trials on German physicians

How did the Nuremberg Doctors' Trials influence the community of German physicians? Did it cause a shock and an upheaval among them, beyond simply the collapse of the Nazi authorities?

The answer to these questions is surprising and disappointing. The body of German physicians after the war showed little interest in the trial and in its outcome. The fact that only twenty physicians were put on trial left the mistaken impression that the majority of physicians in Germany were wholly uninvolved in what took place during the Nazi period. The German Physicians Association eventually published, after some delay, a summary of the trial, edited with commentary by two "observers" it had commissioned, Alexander Mitscherlich and Fred Mielke. A selection of documents submitted to the U.S. court of law were also included. This summary appeared in 1949 in book form, **Wissenschaft ohne Menschlichkeit** (Science Without Humanity), and contained startling revelations. Most of its ten thousand copies sat unread in a warehouse. The book evoked no general response; whereas its American counterpart (mentioned at the end of the last chapter) had some success. Its authors were even accused of slandering and damaging the German medical profession. This hostile avoidance had very damaging consequences, which hampered research into the medical events of the Nazi period to any depth greater than the facts already uncovered by the Nuremberg trials.

Further reading

Trials of War Criminals before the Nuremberg Military Tribunals (the "Medical Case"); Nuremberg, October 1946-April 1949. U.S. Government Printing Office (1949).

T. Childers & J. Caplan (eds.). **Reevaluating the Third Reich.** New York: 1993 (esp. D. Peukert's article, pp. 231-252).

Medizin und Gewissen; 50 Jahre nach dem Nürnberger Ärzteprozeß – Kongreßdokumentation (IPPNW). Frankfurt am Main: Mabuse-Verlag, 1998.

Paul Weindling. **Nazi Medicine and the Nuremberg Trials; From Medical War Crimes to Informed Consent.** Basingstoke: Palgrave-macmillan, 2004

Chapter 14

Medicine and Nazism – an Epilogue

The Nuremberg Doctors' Trials gave many German physicians the feeling that the subject of their criminal cooperation with the Nazis had been resolved. Most of them assumed that the condemnation of the small group in the Nuremberg Trials had exonerated them. Occasionally, stories surfaced of the fruitless search for Josef Mengele, who found refuge and apparently died in South America – and this sufficed for them. After the devastation of the war, physicians in Germany were themselves struggling for survival. Food was scarce and the great desolation of German cities by the Allied bombing had caused a severe shortage of housing. All efforts were channeled into the physical reconstruction of the country. Germany also stood in the shadow of the Cold War between East and West, and in 1949 was divided into two mutually hostile states. The prosecution of the Nazis, including physicians, was no longer a high priority. It was even considered detrimental to the efforts of reconstruction, in which the whole of the German people, including the millions who had supported Hitler and shared his vision of the Third Reich, were meant to participate. The feelings of guilt among some of them probably led them to repress memories of the all-too-recent past.

In schools, almost nothing was taught about the Nazi period. Many teachers in secondary schools had been members of the Nazi party, or held their posts during that period. The majority of them continued teaching after the war. The Ministry of Education, like most government organs, still employed many of the veterans of the Nazi administration. Any changes made only affected the most senior personnel in those offices – and even then only sporadically. The jurist Hans Globke, who had written the commentary on the Nazi racial laws for the Nazi Ministry of the Interior, continued serving in the 1950's as one of the senior advisers to the Federal Chancellery of Konrad Adenauer. East

Germany made extensive propaganda use of this fact to attack its new enemy. Actually, in the East too ex-Nazis served in senior positions; in spite of vaunting itself as being an "anti-Fascist" entity.

One of the senior physicians in East Germany, Prof. Hermann Stieve, retained his high position at the respected Berlin Charité hospital, and was Dean of Medicine at Humboldt University in the city. Many years after his death in 1952, Stieve was exposed as a medical criminal who, for his research purposes, made use of women jailed for their resistance to the Nazi regime. His research included a study of the influence of the emotional pressure to which they were subjected on the eve of their execution and its affect on their menses. Through the efforts of Israeli lawyer Joel Levi and others, who brought to light Stieve's unsavory past, the bronze plaque commemorating him by the main lecture hall of Charité was removed.

Aside from a handful of historians, very few physicians in Germany took interest in the recent past, including the legacy of medical crimes. The memoirs of the celebrated surgeon, Ferdinand Sauerbruch, a collaborator with the Nazi regime (though not a party member himself), a voluminous work of 639 pages published in 1950, only touched upon the criminal actions of Nazi physicians in a meager two or three sentences. He wrote, following the Nuremberg Doctors' Trial: "I can assure that certain physicians, who are certainly not less 'guilty' [*sic*] are continuing their medical profession with impunity." He was right; but he did not content himself with this sentence, adding an instructive (and embarrassing) comment: "I could have cited the names of a dozen such physicians, only that it would not have revived the dead, but would have added some additional victims to the so-questionable process of 'earthly justice'…"

In the West German Physicians Association in the 1950s and 60s, three out of the four heads of the organization had belonged to the Nazi Party. One of them, Hans-Joachim Sewering, had even served in the SS. In 1992, the German delegation to the World Medical Association had the audacity to nominate Dr. Sewering as a candidate for the presidency of the organization, and he was duly selected as president-elect. This step was frustrated only after proof was presented of his personal involvement in the T4 program, including a document he had signed ordering a fourteen-year-old girl to be sent to a "euthanasia" installation. The United States and Israel cooperated in obstructing his final nomination.

In the aftermath of this event, the Israeli Society for the Study of Medicine during the Nazi Period was founded, on the initiative of Prof. Samuel Kottek, lawyer Joel Levi, and the author. Prof. Gerhard Baader volunteered to serve as the Society scientific adviser during its first years, and later on was elected as its head. Additional scholars, such as Prof. Avi Ohry and Dr. Etienne Lepicard, assisted in its activities. The Israeli Society has been a part of the growing movement opposing the world's neglect of such studies, even in the new and democratic Germany.

The generation-long control by former Nazis of the representative body of West German physicians (*"Bundesärztekammer"*) has severely limited the research of medicine during the Nazi period. Its leaders have had a clear personal motive in preventing investigation, including that of persecution of Jewish physicians by their predecessors in the thirties. They have exercised sufficient power to prevent research, even doctoral research, in subjects they have considered too sensitive. Medical students in West Germany have been forced to avoid such delicate issues, for the leaders of the physician organizations had the ability to determine whether and where the graduates could complete their internship.

The heads of these organizations obstructed historical research in other ways; they hermetically sealed off the archives at mental hospitals where "euthanasia" selections were carried out. Under the guise of "safeguarding privacy," they blocked free research and covered the misdeeds of themselves and their colleagues during the Nazi era. Furthermore, their connections with the academic world could prevent the academic advancement of some of the pioneers of historical research into medicine during the Nazi period. Such was the case with Walter Wuttke-Groneberg, the author of the groundbreaking textbook, **Medizin im Nationalsozialismus** (1980), who was accused of "excessive Leftism."

Equally, racist scientists and ex-Nazi physicians continued successfully in postwar Germany. Some of them have even had the insolence to use the fruits of their criminal researches in the Third Reich for their own personal advancement. The race hygienists have undergone a slight mutation: their original occupation, having been tainted, has changed its title to "human genetics."

Fritz Lenz was mentioned previously as one of the three authors of the fundamental book on race hygiene and human heredity. This book was avidly read by Hitler in prison, in 1923, and he extensively quoted it in **Mein Kampf**. In turn, Lenz praised Hitler even before his ascent to power. In 1936, in a new edition of his book that has already become an eugenic and racist classic, Lenz typified the Jews as "a parasitical people". He enrolled as a member of the Nazi Party and as a lecturer on Nazi topics. At the end of the war, the academic career of Lenz was suspended for a while, but in 1949 it was declared that he had been a member of the Nazi Party only through compulsion, and was allowed to continue directing a new institute of human genetics, established on his behalf at the University of Göttingen.

Otmar von Verschuer, Mengele's erstwhile patron, continued his researches after the war as well. His institute in Frankfurt was shut down, but he was appointed in 1953 as professor in Münster, working there until his death in 1969. His son keeps his father's correspondence with Mengele to this day, and refuses to release it for the purpose of research. In 1956, Lenz and von Verschuer, two former Nazis, represented Germany in Copenhagen at the First International Congress of Human Genetics. From that point on, the focus of these congresses shifted to a new subject matter – the influence of nuclear radiation. Other former Nazis, such as Lothar Loeffler, have participated in these conferences.

Nor did the neurologist Julius Hallervorden, who collected the brains of retarded people put to death in 1940 in the "euthanasia" institute at Brandenberg, sit idle after the war. For many years, the brains were preserved in secret in one of the laboratories of the former Kaiser Wilhelm Society. Hallervorden used them for his publications in scientific journals during the war and afterwards. He was careful not to indicate the origin of the brains. His publications achieved their intended purpose, at any rate, and Hallervorden was eventually appointed as a professor at the University of Giessen.

For many years, the Kaiser Wilhelm Society refused to acknowledge any responsibility for the criminal researches carried out under its auspices, making use of the international prestige of the Institute. After the war, its name was changed to Max Planck Society, but this did not signal a major change in its policies. Historians and other scholars, wishing access to it's files from the Nazi period, were flatly refused, up to the last decade.

Pioneers of the new historical research in Germany

In the 1980s, when the geneticist, Benno Müller-Hill, of Cologne dared to examine the war activities of his teachers from the previous generation, he was confronted with many difficulties. In interviews he noted that he was lucky to have received his academic degrees and professorial appointment some years before. Since he was tenured, he could not be harmed professionally. In spite of this, many were angry at him for having dared to break the conspiracy of silence among the scholars of natural sciences.

Müller-Hill was ostracized socially, and his book **Tödliche Wissenschaft** (1984), on the isolation and persecution of Jews, Gypsies, and the mentally ill in Nazi Germany, was virtually banned in Germany, not provoking any public reaction. Its first review was not in Germany, but in the British publication, **Nature**. Only after its translation into English did the book receive a wide circulation – but only outside of Germany. The book contains a wealth of details about the shameful involvement of the national research body, the *"Deutsche Forschungsgemeinschaft"* [DFG] (the German science community), still active today, in financing and carrying out dubious studies in the Nazi period, some of which were openly criminal. For instance, a study on "specific proteins," planned to be held using human guinea-pigs in Auschwitz under the scientific direction of Josef Mengele, was financed generously by the DFG.

In its conclusion, Müller-Hill's book raised the fear that similar dubious methods could be used to control the human genetic code. The separation that had already been made in the Third Reich between Science and Morality, between the deed and its consequences, was a crucial motif of Müller-Hill's book about the past, which also serves as a warning for the future.

The program of "euthanasia" was the only aspect of Nazi medicine where new discoveries were made in the first generation after the war. Events taking place after the official end of the T4 program, in summer 1941, received special attention. As a result, physicians and nurses who put psychiatric patients to death, children especially, in what was known as "wild euthanasia," were put on trial – since it was clear to everybody that this was a case of private initiative and excessive zeal, even by Nazi standards. Such was the case, for one example, of Dr. Walter Gross, who served throughout the war in the children's ward of a Vienna psychiatric hospital, and even after the war used organs taken from the bodies of murdered children for his own research. In 1950 he received a mere two years imprisonment, and a year later was pardoned.

In the 1950s and 60s, relatives of the victims of the T4 program and people who had been sterilized and had survived the war appealed to the authorities for recognition of, and compensation for, their suffering. Their requests were rejected. They did provoke a new interest in the subject, however, which has grown thanks to people such as the social worker, Ernst Klee. He knew some of the victims and was a pioneer of the historical research of the subject.

Occasionally, some nurses who had worked under the physicians in the death institutes came forward to give evidence. Thus it became possible in the 1960s and 70s to try additional doctors for the medical murders, and these trials provoked a stronger public resonance than previously. One of the trials, which gained much interest, dealt with the psychiatric clinic in Eglfing-Haar, near Munich. Here, and in other institutions for the mentally ill, some patients were murdered even after the Nazi surrender!

These few cases aside, most criminal physicians, and not only those involved in the "euthanasia" program, continued to practice their profession undisturbed for many years. The SS doctor, Aribert Heim, who was active in the Mauthausen, Buchenwald and Sachsenhausen concentration camps, is such an example. Heim murdered victims by injecting phenol directly into their hearts, among other criminal acts. After the war he had a thriving medical practice in a small town near Frankfurt without even having to change his identity. Finally he was forced to go into hiding in the 1960s, after Eichmann's capture. Only then did the German police issue an arrest warrant for him. He fled from Germany, and was held in Spain in 2005, after two generations had passed since the time of his crimes. Because of his advanced age, and some doubts about his identity many think he will never face justice.

The slackness in prosecuting the criminals of Nazi medicine had an unforeseen result: the confidence of many German patients, psychiatric patients in particular, was badly shaken in the postwar period. A decided decline in hospitalization became evident,[1] as was the reduced inclination of medical students to specialize in psychiatry.

The turnabout in the German medical establishment and its implications for research of the Nazi period

Only from the 1980s, could a gradual change be noticed in Germany with regards to the research into medical crimes. The main reason for this was the change of generations taking place within the medical establishment. The new leaders of the physicians' organizations were too young to have been former Nazis. Furthermore, a new generation of young physicians and historians emerged – partly drawn from and influenced by the students' rebellion of the 1960s – which made it its mission to expose the deeds of their fathers. Archives were gradually opened. Scholars of repute, like Gerhard Baader and Berlin physician Christian Pross, organized conferences dealing with uncovering the past.

Books by well-known Western scholars on the subject were now being translated into German. Such titles included: **The Nazi Doctors; Medical Killing and the Psychology of Genocide** by Robert Jay Lifton, the Jewish psychiatrist who interviewed SS doctors and imprisoned physicians, and the study by Michael Kater, **Doctors under Hitler**, on the popularity of the Nazi doctrine among German physicians. Younger scholars, such as Götz Aly and Michael Hubenstorf (who now lives in Vienna and researches the crimes of Nazi doctors there), were gradually swelling the previously small numbers of historians who dealt with this subject.

The researchers of the new generation do not stay cloistered in ivory towers. Most of them are actively involved in the present with the implications of their studies of the past. Through their initiative and pressure, a number of universities and research institutes have disposed

---

1   The decline of psychiatric cases was partially due to the physical annihilation of
     many potential patients in the Nazi "euthanasia."

of tissue samples from their stores, which had been removed from the bodies of victims and were sent from the death camps by Mengele and his confreres. Some of these samples, kept in formalin all those years as instruction material, have been buried in a suitable manner in the last few years. The University of Tübingen used the occasion to hold a conference on the subject. This and other institutions have issued public apologies to the victims of medical experimentation and have tried to learn the lessons of history for the benefit of the future. Too many other places, however, have not held any expiatory actions, and to this day suspected anatomical samples and teaching aids remain. Thus, an anatomical textbook, inspired by the Austrian professor, Eduard Pernkopf, suspected of having illustrated his atlas through the use of tissue samples taken from the bodies of Jewish prisoners is still in use. Despite the efforts of scholars such as William Seidelmann to expose Pernkopf's transgressions, all that was finally done was to delete from the illustrations the swastika decorated signatures of the atlas artists who had been members of the SS.

Certain scientists have acted in the opposite way: editors of prestigious publications, such as the **New England Journal of Medicine**, forbade any mention of the results of studies carried out through suspect methodology, no matter what the contribution to medical knowledge might be. Bodies such as the Max Planck Society (the former Kaiser Wilhelm Society) were finally persuaded in the nineties to cooperate with historical research – and financed the research into their past during the dark period. This study, undertaken by scholars of renown such as the British Paul Weindling, has already born fruit, and continues to be published in a number of volumes.

Combining study of the past with bio-ethics

The new historians in German faculties of medicine consider it a privilege and necessity to teach the history of the Nazi period combined with medical ethics. These days, it is a compulsory subject of study, of special urgency in the light of developments – not only in Germany – in the realm of genetics and modern medicine. Once more, questions dealing with the human genetic heredity are on the agenda, this time supported by real science – the uncovering of the secrets of the DNA and the human genome. Such research has created the future possibility of being able to influence the characteristics and appearance of the newborn by means of genetic consultation of some sort. The nature of this consultation and its substance – whether private or "official" and established – is controversial, and rightly so. On the one hand, there is a justified desire to protect the individual's freedom and right of choice. On the other hand, there are potential dangers to the social fabric – from determining the sex of the unborn fetus, which may have grave demographic implications. In China and India, advances in pre-natal technologies have led to millions of female fetuses being aborted. "Ordering the newborn" with preferred eye, skin or hair color may reinforce stereotypes and reward racism.

In our generation, new dilemmas have emerged, born from medicine's ability to extend life through artificial means. This is a question of bio-ethics involving moral decisions about the value of life and what right the physician has to end it when the patient suffers and is unable to derive any enjoyment from his life.

The history of medicine under the Nazis is a warning-call about euthanasia and similar issues, to prevent physicians from sliding down a slippery and dangerous downward road, as the Nazi doctors did. One is reminded of the prophetic warning of Julius Moses in 1932, about physicians imbued with Nazi racism becoming murderers, a prophecy fulfilled with catastrophic results for humanity. We have to learn from this history that many issues need the contribution of different disciplines of study. We must not relegate sole authority in such areas to the medical establishment alone. The training of medical students must broaden their horizons, lest future physicians be faced with the intoxicating sense of omnipotence. This intoxication tempted doctors to abandon their values and led also to the medicalization of the Holocaust. Engaging with ethics in medical instruction in the university environment and combining such study with lessons gained from the recent past is of crucial importance.

In some chapters of this book, we have witnessed the attempts of Jewish physicians to maintain the principles of traditional medical ethics even in hellish circumstances. Their efforts and fortitude were generally of little avail; but there are many of them whose very rectitude and behavior in such adversity may serve as an instructive model for the proper way of dealing with bio-ethical questions of the present and the future.

Further reading

Medicine, Ethics and the Third Reich; Historical and Contemporary Issues (edited by John J. Michalczyk). Kansas City: Sheed and Ward, 1994.

Medizin im "Dritten Reich" (edited by Johanna Bleker and Norbert Jachertz). Köln: Deutscher Ärzte-Verlag, 1993 (2. ed.).

Benno Müller-Hill. **Murderous Science; Elimination by scientific selection of Jews, Gypsies, and others, Germany 1933-1945.** Oxford, New York, Tokyo: Oxford University Press, 1988.

Index